LET GO OF EMOTIONAL OVER-EATING AND LOVE YOUR FOOD

LET GO OF EMOTIONAL OVER-EATING AND LOVE YOUR FOOD

A Five-Point Plan for Success

Arlene B. Englander

ROWMAN & LITTLEFIELD
Lanham • Boulder • New York • London

Published by Rowman & Littlefield
An imprint of The Rowman & Littlefield Publishing Group, Inc.
4501 Forbes Boulevard, Suite 200, Lanham, Maryland 20706
www.rowman.com

Unit A, Whitacre Mews, 26-34 Stannary Street, London SE11 4AB

British Library Cataloguing in Publication Information Available

Library of Congress Cataloging-in-Publication Data

Names: Englander, Arlene B., author.
Title: Let go of emotional overeating and love your food : a five-point plan for success / Arlene B. Englander.
Description: Lanham : Rowman & Littlefield, [2018] | Includes bibliographical references and index.
Identifiers: LCCN 2018001633 (print) | LCCN 2017060903 (ebook) | ISBN 9781538111192 (cloth : alk. paper) | ISBN 9781538111208 (electronic)
Subjects: LCSH: Compulsive eating. | Food habits—Psychological aspects.
Classification: LCC RC552.C65 E54 2018 (ebook) | LCC RC552.C65 (print) | DDC 616.85/26—dc23
LC record available at https://lccn.loc.gov/2018001633

♾ ™ The paper used in this publication meets the minimum requirements of American National Standard for Information Sciences Permanence of Paper for Printed Library Materials, ANSI/NISO Z39.48-1992.

Printed in the United States of America

To my loving husband; my darling daughter; and my parents, two of the kindest people I have ever known.

CONTENTS

INTRODUCTION

Is this book for you? *Let Go of Emotional Overeating and Love Your Food: A Five-Point Plan for Success* is for you if you feel entrapped by emotional eating. It's for you if you ever leave a table feeling stuffed both physically with food and psychologically with self-hate. It's for you if you're drawn to food when stressed, depressed, or anxious and sense there's a better way to self-soothe, "but what?" It's for you if you've yo-yo dieted for decades—fantasizing about forbidden foods until a diet-ending binge replaces pounds that were lost and adds more.

This book is for you if you'd like to find new freedom. It's for you if you'd like to be able to eat whatever you like, savor your food, and stop just at the point of satisfaction without feeling full. It's for you if you'd like to feel in control of life's stress instead of controlled by it. It's for you if you'd like to enjoy your days and evenings to the utmost, instead of abusing or obsessing about food.

It's hard to gauge to how many of us this applies, but if weight alone is any indication, the numbers are high. Most Americans need to lose weight and know the only way to do so is by eating less and moving more. There's only one problem: they can do neither. For many, compulsive overeating is the issue that keeps them from getting to a healthy weight and staying there.

How did we arrive at this dangerous health epidemic? As early as 1999, *American Demographics* published the article "Getting Bigger All the Time"—a title that certainly proved prophetic (!), reporting that

- 54 percent of all Americans clean their plates even when they're full
- 39 percent eat when they see food
- 20 percent eat when depressed
- 19 percent continue to eat when stuffed[1]

Does any of this feel familiar?

While we don't have stats on how many of us eat emotionally, a Pew Report from 2006 indicates that six in ten Americans say they eat more than they should, either often (17 percent) or sometimes (42 percent).[2]

And according to the Centers for Disease Control and Prevention (CDC), as of 2014, 37.9 percent of adults twenty years of age and older were obese, and 70.7 percent were either overweight or obese, while in an equally disturbing trend, 9.4 percent of two- to five-year-olds, 17.4 percent of six- to eleven-year-olds, and 20.6 percent of adolescents were in the heaviest category of weight.[3]

If you can relate, then clearly you have company. And having "been there and done that" in the past, I can, too. Yes, this is a prevalent problem. But there are answers.

Let Go of Emotional Overeating and Love Your Food is written expressly to help you if you're trying to change the behaviors listed above. It offers specific strategies on how to savor food and be satisfied with less, minimize stress, maximize enjoyment, and make healthy habits like exercise really happen. Most important, the book's main focus is teaching you how to stop eating when you're just exactly full. This habit can be learned and you'll love the results.

The basic theme is simple. By developing an awareness of what constitutes compulsive overeating and by learning how to eat in a more pleasure-oriented, self-regulated manner, you'll not only enjoy food more but will also gain control. An additional emphasis is on creating and maintaining a better balance between the joys derived from food and life.

A licensed psychotherapist for more than twenty years and a former emotional overeater, I include, when appropriate, case illustrations and personal experiences. I also use humor and anecdotes as an effective teaching tool.

Having earned an MBA, I also incorporate numerous devices to help you "operationalize" the advice given, such as acronyms for mealtime techniques and for tracking your progress in following the plan every day. A unique aspect to this program is the "one-minute monitor" that is anchored into the reader's mind by two quick questions, the first of which includes a four-letter acronym, making it possible, daily, hourly, and instantaneously, to review and tweak one's efforts in following this plan, and the second refers to a joke and a play on words, reminding the reader of point number 5 in the plan:

Are you doing what's best for your "SELF"?
Are you a "light" eater?

Also unique is the book's emphasis on encouraging enjoyment so that this is a plan you'll want to pursue permanently!

As a former emotional overeater myself, I know how painful those experiences can be. And it's often undetected. I completed an entire course of psychoanalysis without realizing that "everybody" doesn't obsess about food all day, eat voraciously for several days in a row, and then survive on coffee or Diet Coke and cigarettes to compensate for the calories for the next few days, or suffer the deprivation of restrictive diets that only end in a binge. Having been entrapped in that cycle, it's gratifying to lead others to new freedom.

I hope you join me on this journey to moving past emotional eating and to getting more joy out of food and life. It's a journey I've made and I feel grateful to be able help you, too.

1

"LOVE MY FOOD?!"

"Love my food?," you may be asking. "Isn't my problem that I love food too much?" These are questions I frequently encounter when I present a *Love Your Food*® seminar or hold my first session with a client. You may also find it hard to believe that the key to the issues you and most emotional overeaters have with food is that you don't enjoy it enough!

"But I love to eat!" is a frequent response. "I'm always cleaning the plate, whether I'm hungry or not, and it's hard for me to stop snacking on all the sweet, rich foods I adore but know I shouldn't have."

This book is about the difference between truly tasting and savoring food—enjoying the magnificent experience of eating—as opposed to compulsively finishing whatever is on your plate or snacking due to stress.

Yes, food is to be loved! But that's an attitude that many of us—especially those of us with a dieting mentality—find shocking. "How will I ever be able to control my weight if I allow myself to love my food?" you may be asking. The beauty of the *Love Your Food*® approach is that by really tasting and experiencing food and being there in the moment as you eat, you'll be able to find not only true enjoyment, but also true control.

The ideas I'll be sharing are based on my work with clients for more than twenty years as a licensed psychotherapist, augmented by my own experiences as a compulsive overeater. I've learned a lot by observing others, and myself. It's wonderful to no longer eat compulsively—to be able to eat whatever I like, whenever I choose, and to look forward to each new meal (when I remember to think about food) with excitement. It's great to be free from dieting yet still to be slim and fit.

What's the difference between my current way of eating and my habits in the past? One of the most important observations I've made, both personally and professionally, is that there's a key difference between compulsive eating and eating in a healthy, truly satisfying way. Normal eating is different both in *quantity* and *quality*.

To make this more understandable, let's look at an analogy. Were we to ask an alcoholic whether he or she really loved wine, the answer would probably be a resounding "Yes." However, were we to ask this same person to describe in detail the exact taste, texture, and body of a vintage and to differentiate one from another, we'd get a vague answer, if any. What's important to this unfortunate individual is not the experience of drinking the beverage, but only its ability to produce a numbing effect. If one can't take true pleasure in life, there's little joy to be found in wine. The latter becomes only a pitiful attempt to escape pain.

The wine connoisseur, on the other hand, is quintessentially aware of every aspect of the experience when tasting a vintage. As we watch, we can almost sense the expert's appreciation while imbibing and lingering lovingly over every moment. Wine is taken seriously and savored as part of a balanced repertoire of one of life's many passions.

What we're seeking to achieve while eating is a similar level of awareness and balance; a sense of being in the moment that will help us enjoy our food but control our intake. In addition, extending that awareness to other aspects of our lives will reap equally great rewards.

Having contrasted the alcoholic with the wine connoisseur, we're ready to look at a concept that has helped my clients—as well as me—in conquering emotional overeating.

Emotional overeating is eating neither to satisfy hunger nor for enjoyment, but in a desperate attempt to distract oneself from painful thoughts and feelings.

Loving food is the polar opposite of abusing it. Unfortunately, most Americans have a love–hate relationship with food. We both crave it and fear it, an attitude fostered by the dieting industry. Feeling that a number of the foods we like are forbidden, many of us tend to overeat them whenever they're available.

Perhaps the thought of trying a new approach is scary—even one emphasizing the importance of taking pleasure in food and life. Perhaps you've tried diets and feel you've "failed." Perhaps you've attempted other programs but feel you've floundered because there was no way to pinpoint your progress in practicing new habits. I know because I've been there—with clients and myself. In the next chapter we'll look at how diets help create rather than cure food compulsions, so the "solution" fails, not you. Later you'll learn how to ask yourself two questions—one containing a simple acronym anchoring four of the habits you'll need to adopt and another introducing the fifth point in the five-point plan. These two questions together make a "one-minute monitor" you can use daily to track and tweak your efforts. You'll also learn a second easy-to-remember acronym so that every meal will be an opportunity to savor your food and stop just at the point of satisfaction, a skill that will eventually become instinctive.

Sadly, many new clients come to me complaining that they've been "good" that week or "bad." They blame themselves for having a "bad" day or week until I emphasize that being good or bad has no relevance to our work. Blaming or labeling ourselves is one of the habits causing our pain and which we'll learn to control when we learn to lessen stress. Since compulsive eating is an attempt to distract oneself from pain, anything creating emotional pain contributes to emotional eating.

Does this pattern of self-hate feel familiar? If so, rest assured that by tuning in to these thoughts and their origins, we'll turn them around in a caring, compassionate way. When we focus on stress you'll learn new habits of soothing yourself sans food—habits that will become instantaneous and even fun! You'll be free to find more pleasure—not just an escape from pain—in food and life.

Awareness is a skill we must embrace and enhance for any program of behavioral change to succeed. It's important to become aware of situations during which you eat too much, as well as times when a meal is satisfying and you're able to stop eating just at the inception of fullness. Adopting a compassionate, accepting awareness of our behavior as we begin to change will make it easier to learn and grow.

Begin by noticing the eating styles of others. There's a visible difference in the behavior of those with healthy—as opposed to unhealthy—relationships with food. Watch people as they eat. Do they hunch over the table, wolfing down their food as if afraid that someone might steal it away? Or do they sit back comfortably and show an observable appreciation of every bite? Are they multitasking during the meal, hardly eyeing what they're eating, giving almost total attention to a screen, or two, or three?!

The next time you're in a restaurant compare and contrast the habits of people you observe. Notice differences between those who appear to be compulsive overeaters and those who don't. Remember that body size can be deceptive. People of normal weight can nevertheless have an eating disorder.

After a while certain patterns will emerge. You'll see that those who seem fitter tend, on average, to take smaller portions, eat more slowly, and savor their food. What's almost invisible, however, is the attitude that naturally slim, intuitive eaters often share. Though food is important to them and they appear to enjoy it, they're active and involved in many productive and pleasurable pursuits. They seem to be savoring the conversation and pleasant surroundings as much or more than what they're eating. They may love food, but they love their lives more.

Consider this fable of a woman embarking alone on her first cruise, a weekend excursion. On Saturday morning she arrived in the dining room at nine o'clock and ordered juice and an omelet. At ten she ordered pancakes. By eleven she was sipping coffee and munching on a pastry. At noon she was drinking a refill as the lunch crowd entered. At one in the afternoon she ordered soup and a salad and an entrée. At two she tried a second entrée, then had dessert. Following several cups of coffee and a sampling of other treats it was five o'clock and dinner began. After dining at length, she returned to her cabin at ten to sleep. The following day she repeated this pattern. On arriving home she called a friend to chat about the trip. When asked about the voyage, she answered, "It was a nice cruise, but there was just one problem. They only feed you one meal a day!"

This lady truly "missed the boat" (pun intended!) in terms of taking true pleasure in food and life. As this humorous anecdote illustrates, focusing on food alone won't help us control unnecessary eating. Without placing added pleasures on the plate of life, we'll suffer the same disappointment as the tragicomic traveler above.

Let's look back for a moment at our definition for emotional overeating—*eating neither for enjoyment nor to satisfy hunger, but in a desperate attempt to distract oneself from painful thoughts and feelings.* If that speaks to you, you're not alone. In countless sessions, seminars, and other settings I've seen people nod their heads in recognition.

But focusing only on the "problem" is counterproductive and not in the style of the positive, solution-oriented work I do. Try it. If you've worked on improving your tennis or golf, for example, you know that you need an awareness of what's amiss with your swing. But if you focus solely on what's wrong, what happens? If you're a tennis player, try telling yourself, "I'd better not fault" the next time you serve and see what happens! A fault's inevitable! On the other hand, thinking, "Hit it in!" is often helpful.

Picking a pattern of thought or behavior that's positive and practicing it until it's a habit is what's most helpful in achieving change. So in *Let Go of Emotional Overeating and Love Your Food* we'll occasionally glance back at the concept of compulsive overeating, but the emphasis will always be on eating and living in a healthier, more enjoyment-oriented way.

The best advice I can give to you right now is this: ask yourself what, in addition to eating, would be fun and allow yourself to do it!

One of the most popular courses at Harvard was the basis for a book titled *Happier* by Tal Ben-Shahar.[1] Every week hundreds of students listened to his lectures to learn something that seemed novel to a number of those high achievers—the importance of pleasure in their lives. But Professor Ben-Shahar wasn't preaching hedonism, a meaningless escape that often masks despair. In his course on positive psychology he emphasized the importance of finding meaning and pleasure in our lives so that we can find a balance that is truly satisfying.

When I was working in corporate health promotion and studying for my master's in business administration at New York University, I took a course in international business relations. The professor, wise, worldly, and in his fifties, was teaching a class containing predominantly twenty-five-year-old middle management corporate types—aspiring "captains of industry." To highlight the richness and complexity of other cultures, the professor spoke of an evening in Japan, where, with a group of fellow businessmen, he'd visited a geisha house and spent a wonderful evening drinking tea and singing songs. The males in the class, incredulous that this was all he'd done and remembered it fondly, responded with a chorus of hoots, to which the teacher replied, "When was the last time you sang?" A somber silence fell upon the room.

When was the last time *you* sang? Or danced? Or acted silly? Ask yourself what pursuits you've postponed that might bring you pleasure. Many of my clients take up sports, sign up for adult education classes, learn new hobbies or crafts, or resume old ones—the list is long. When we allow ourselves to become fully engaged in meaningful and pleasurable activities we achieve a state of "flow" whereby we're blissfully in the moment and time stands still as it goes by. This experience is wonderfully fulfilling. We may feel it when we are with a loved one, engaged in a sport, playing a musical instrument, doing work we find truly meaningful, enjoying a craft, or, if you happen to be me, doing all of the above and many more, including the writing of the words I'm sharing with you now!

Is it puzzling to begin our work together talking about pleasure? Does that seem "selfish" in a negative way? Ask yourself this—if you'd grown up in a home with people who were happier, more fulfilled, and really with you "in the moment," would your life have been better or worse? Sadly, many of my clients say their obsession with food renders them uncomfortable with themselves and others. Mothers are distracted from their children by self-hate because they overate at their last meal and worry about what and when they will eat next. Twenty-something women can't cook for their boyfriends for fear they'll eat compulsively before, during, and after the meal. Persons of all ages turn down social evenings to remain alone at home and binge. Only when we're comfortable with ourselves and "in the moment" can we be there in an empathic, loving way for others.

Why all this seriousness about liking, even loving, what we do in *Let Go of Emotional Overeating and Love Your Food*? How can we even be talking about *fun* in the context of curing compulsive eating and achieving weight control? It's essential, is the answer, because if what we do isn't pleasurable it won't be permanent. Without pleasure you may change your behavior in the short term but not in the long term, nor for a lifetime—which is what counts.

Take a moment now to visualize yourself the way you'd like to be. Ponder what would give you the most pleasure about being in control of your eating and being the healthiest and fittest you can be. Create a fantasy that's truly fantastic—one that turns you on to feeling good and doing what's best for yourself—while we work together to make it real.

For example, if you're a tennis player and would savor the thought of walking up to the net at the start of a match looking fit and like a daunting contender, use that thought as well as the appeal of the added energy you'd have to get to the ball and play well. But don't require that you win every game, not only in fantasy but also in real life. If so, you've forgotten the fun and you're in for trouble.

Doug, whom I worked with early in my career, was thirty-five, divorced, and a salesman of luxury cars. He was five ten, weighed 250 pounds, and stated that he desperately wanted to change his habit of almost constant compulsive overeating whenever he was home. His main objective in working with me, however, as I later found out, pertained to his frustration with his girlfriend of four years who insisted on seeing other men. He expected that once he lost weight this would stop and she'd accept his proposal of marriage. Within a year he'd learned to limit his excessive overeating, was exercising, and had lost fifty pounds. But when his girlfriend's behavior didn't budge he became furious first with her and then with me (!). It took a lot of work to prevent him from resuming past patterns and regaining all the weight and more.

The takeaway lesson here is to choose objectives that are within your control. So visualize yourself having fun, but keep your focus on how good *you* feel about *yourself* and the positive work *you've* done—be it at a party, on the beach, engaging in a sport, speaking at a conference, playing with your kids—whatever, wherever, with whomever.

Does fun still seem far-fetched as a key component of a "self-help" plan? It shouldn't. If food and only food is your main source of pleasure and your primary strategy for soothing pain, you'll always have issues with compulsive overeating.

Here's a story of a "single-session cure." Leslie, whose children had recently moved away from home for college, came to see me complaining that she tended to eat compulsively between three and five in the afternoon. Midafternoon was when she was alone at home with unstructured time. She'd been snacking, she came to realize, to distract herself from boredom—best described by Theodore Isaac Rubin, MD, as a form of self-hate, anger we aim toward ourselves because we aren't utilizing our full potential.[2] So Leslie and I brainstormed about hobbies, interests, and opportunities she might explore, all with the goal of adding purpose and pleasure to her life. End result? She called me to cancel her next session, phoning to tell me she was volunteering in the afternoons for the local cultural council, loved it, and no longer compulsively overate. My unbooked hour aside, I see that as a success!

Let's return to your visualization. What are you doing and how do you feel? Some clients say "confident." Others say "beautiful," "attractive," "sexy," "strong," or "secure." Here's a secret: there isn't any reason you can't start to feel this way right now! "How can I?" new clients frequently ask. "I'm too fat."

This cruel self-blame is self-induced pain we'll work later to eradicate. For now, just keep in mind that your current weight is most closely connected with who you've been in the *past*—your habits, home, the society you inhabit. Accepting who you are *today* will help you evolve into who you'd like to be *tomorrow*.

Not long ago I received a call from Amanda, a young woman who hadn't spoken to her mother for a decade. She had married and now, as a new mom of twins, wanted to try to revive the relationship. She felt this way in spite of many years of near-estrangement and her insistence that she'd been abandoned. Her mother, Marie, flew in from a distance, arriving early for our first session with a very different picture of their past and a stack of angry emails spanning several years that she wished to make the main point of our meeting. Glancing at the stack of pages, I suggested we make the best of the present moment, rather than looking back in anger or mistrustfully toward the future. Before we met with Amanda I pointed toward my window to the name on the boat moored nearby. Marie looked out, understood, and rushed downstairs to hide the heap of papers. What's the name of the boat? "Seas the Day."

Let's seize the day ourselves and embark on this plan for letting go of emotional eating—permanently and pleasurably. Enjoy the journey!

2

DIETS DO WORK—TO CAUSE COMPULSIVE OVEREATING AND BINGEING!

Since you've read this far you're most likely fed up (pun intended) with dieting and searching for a new approach to change your eating yet control your weight. But the thought of change may seem scary, even sinful. Diets seem to be everywhere—promoted online, on TV, in print, and in conversation.

We live in a rapidly changing, unpredictable world. While many of us feel concerned about our country, our world, our economy, our families, and our jobs, we're also barraged by marketing-driven messages about food and weight. Though not a physical attack on our personas, they can certainly damage our psyche. These are the messages, sometimes subtle, at other times direct, that say that if you're a female in this society you can never be too young, too slim, too successful, too busy, or even too busty! If you're male, you can eliminate a few of the above expectations, adding on, however, the pressure to be tall, sporting big biceps and well-defined abs.

Given the stress of our high-paced, tension-packed, high-tech world, the allure of easy solutions to emotional eating and achieving healthy weight is highly appealing. We long for solutions that are quick and simple, either by eating one food but not another; severely restricting food intake on some days but not others; or by taking a supplement that works miraculously and immediately, requiring neither effort nor discipline on our part. The huge appeal of schemes to get thin quick is rivaled in size only by the financial awards available to those who promote swift and simplistic solutions.

Years ago, as a fledgling clinician *and* a compulsive overeater and dieter, I interviewed at a firm offering weight loss via strict calorie counting and the consumption of only packaged foods. The owner, a portly man, first questioned me about my experience and interest in the weight loss field. Then he asked if I had questions about him and the position. Finally, he looked at me purposefully and posed what I perceived to be the "make or break" query of the interview. "Tell me, young lady, what do you think we are here for?" Faltering for a moment, I responded uncertainly, "To help people?" "No!" he shouted, his face turning red with rage as he rose to his feet, "We're here for one reason and one reason only—to make money!" The interview was over. I didn't get the job, nor did I want it. I was fortunate, I feel, to have moved forward, training and working at reputable organizations, developing the concepts I'm sharing with you now.

The desperation of dieters and the potential profits for promoters contribute to the constant stream of food proscriptions and prescriptions popping up for the past few decades. The omnipresence of these programs and their successful marketing to the public has created an illusion (or more accurately, a delusion) that's widely held in this society.

What is this myth? It's the belief that there are two types of people on the planet—those prone to be overweight and therefore doomed to dieting, versus others blessed to be naturally slim and able to eat whatever they choose. If letting go of diets and the dieting mentality is scary to you, it's possible your belief in this myth is contributing to your concern.

Several years ago, I was attending an all-day conference for teachers and therapists and was still a bit sleepy during breakfast when I spied a platter of pastries. Spontaneously, I said, "Those look delicious!," to which the bearer of the bounty defensively declared, "It's my last day of vacation, so I can eat whatever I want!" Unthinkingly, I responded, "I always do." After looking me over she answered, "I've one word for you, and I won't say it out loud here!" as she turned abruptly, beating an angry retreat.

Little did she realize I would have loved to talk to her about my past dieting debacles, as well as impart how I've learned to now savor small quantities of whatever I like. But people like the "pastry lady" have been so immersed in the marketing-driven mythology we spoke of earlier that it's hard for them to believe that people can learn new, healthier habits. They're incapable of imagining a life free of food fear—a life in which every day is a vacation from overly restrictive eating.

A growing number of us in the field of psychotherapy, psychology, nutrition, and science are arriving at the realization that strict, restrictive diets are often counterproductive. Charlotte N. Markey, a psychology professor at Rutgers and an eating and dieting researcher, wrote a brilliant piece titled "Don't Diet." Markey offers this:

> My advice as a psychologist and researcher who focuses on weight control: Do not diet. Do not cut out groups of foods or cut calories. Do not try to eat very little or deprive yourself. Such strategies backfire because of psychological effects that every dieter is all too familiar with: intense cravings for foods you have eliminated, bingeing on junk food after falling off the wagon, an intense preoccupation with food. A growing body of research shows why these tendencies undermine most people's diet efforts and confirms that the way around these pitfalls is moderation. Making small changes to your eating patterns, ones you can build on slowly over time, is truly the best pathway to lasting weight loss. Although you may have heard this message of moderation before, the evidence is finally too overwhelming to ignore.[1]

You may still feel skeptical, exposed as you are to the influence of a mammoth marketing machine that has generated a $40 billion dieting industry. But research shows that 95 percent of dieters regain whatever weight they've lost and more within a year. And after five years, 98 percent of dieters regain their lost weight plus ten pounds.[2] Nonetheless, dieters continue to persecute and punish themselves rather than critique the painful process by which they've tried to control their weight. As Jackie Gleason aptly put it, "The best day of any diet is the second day, because by then you're off it!"

So if dieting doesn't work, how do we "undiet"? The clue to a new way of eating and living is found in the word *diet* itself. To *diet* is to *die* a little, turning off our awareness of hunger and satiety and of exactly what foods in which amounts we need and crave.

The reverse is a process of expanding awareness—starting with the way we react to all we see, hear, and actually sense in any way. For example, the next time you hear someone raving about the latest diet, look at their appearance. Compulsive overeaters come in various shapes and sizes, but the most vocal proponents of restrictive eating rarely look as fit as you'd ultimately like to be. In other words, to put it bluntly, check out the size of those presenting the most powerful sales pitch to their friends.

Now begin to expand your inner awareness by exploring how dieting has let you down personally, compounding the problems you were desperately using it to solve. To do so, let's look at some of the most common reactions to dieting. Think of the last time you seriously restricted your eating, counting every calorie, weighing yourself often as you anxiously checked the scale for results that would merit your misery. Here's a list of reactions—by no means all-inclusive—based on feedback from clients as well as myself:

- A sense of deprivation
- Irritability
- Gnawing hunger
- Recurrent thoughts, bordering on obsessions, about forbidden foods
- Envy of others who seem uniquely able to eat whatever they wish
- Desire to binge on "forbidden" foods
- Guilt and self-loathing when diet is "broken"
- Boredom, bordering on depression due to limited, repetitive choice of foods
- Add your own here!

Yes, this is certainly a depressing scenario. One of life's greatest pleasures seems prohibited. In fact, our sense of taste and the delectation we derive from it is central to our satisfaction in life—so much so that research indicates that people who permanently lose their ability to taste may become severely depressed, even suicidal.

As we continue to explore our awareness of life while dieting and of the influences supporting our belief that this is the sole way to control weight, let's revisit a key concept in our work, one mentioned earlier in chapter 1—the definition of emotional overeating.

Emotional overeating can be defined as eating neither for enjoyment nor for the satisfaction of hunger, but in a desperate attempt to distract oneself from painful thoughts and feelings.

Is there anything here that seems ironic? Think about it for a moment. Isn't the list above replete with the types of thoughts and feelings any right-minded person would chose to escape in almost any possible way? And for the chronic compulsive overeater, which form of escape would be their "substance of choice"? You've got it! Food! This is the perfect scenario for the continuation and even creation of compulsive overeating and bingeing. The "cure" for the condition actually helps create it!

To further explore how this happens, examine the illustration in figure 2.1, which shows how dieting and binge eating become a vicious cycle—a downward spiral in which we feel frustrated, stressed, angry, anxious, or depressed; choose to overeat, feel worse, eat more, feel even worse, ad infinitum.

Given this scenario it's only logical, as noted above, that, according to Anorexia Nervosa & Related Eating Disorders (ANRED), 98 percent of dieters regain all the weight they've lost plus ten pounds within five years.[3] Most diets have a binge at the end of it.

This is how the above syndrome operates. A client named Suzanne, a stunning brunette businesswoman, suffered from binge eating and bulimia. In one of our sessions Suzanne recalled an experience on a business trip when a man seated next to her on an airplane asked her if she'd like a few jelly beans. After eating several she had some more and before she gave it conscious thought had finished the whole box. Annoyed at herself and her "sin," she continued to overeat later that evening even to the point of painfulness. Her explanation was sadly prophetic. "Once I'd had one jelly bean I felt I'd blown it, so why not go for broke?"

This go-for-broke philosophy is a typical response to the deprivation of dieting. Once restrictions are broken, the dieter, now labeling herself a "cheater," feels she may as well go all the way. Feeling the pain of the negative label, and desperate to flee that pain, she then resorts to numbing out by overeating the forbidden food or foods.

What's especially sad about this scenario is that little or no enjoyment is derived. I know this personally. I obtain far more pleasure today consuming one mid-sized cookie, slowly savored, as I sit and sip a small

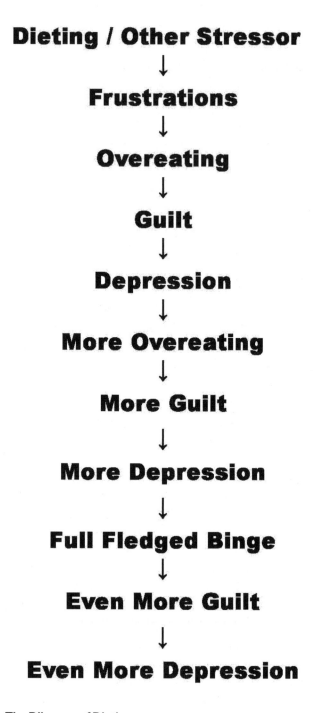

Figure 2.1.   The Dilemma of Dieting

glass of skim milk, than I used to experience standing up while wolfing down a whole box. As I relax and appreciate the taste and texture of each bite, I might reminisce about a similar snack indulged with my friends on wintry Friday nights, arriving in Vermont at almost midnight, feeling tired after the day's work and the long drive, but also excited about the upcoming weekend of skiing and socializing.

This experience of being relaxed and in the moment—pleasantly aware of oneself and one's environment while really tasting and enjoying food—is totally antithetical to bingeing. It's this "in the moment" awareness that you'll need to discover and encourage within yourself in order to let go of emotional eating and feel the way you want to feel.

In his excellent book *The Power of Habit*, Charles Duhigg, a Pulitzer prize–winning investigative reporter and a graduate of Harvard Business School, puts his wits to work at uncovering the mystique of habits. Describing what happens he writes,

> This process within our brain is a three-step loop. First there is a *cue*, a trigger that tells your brain to go into automatic mode and which habit to use. Then there is the *routine*, which can be physical or mental or emotional. Finally, there is a *reward*, which helps your brain figure out if this reward is worth remembering for the future. Over time, this loop—cue, routine, reward; cue, routine, reward— becomes more and more automatic. The cue and reward become intertwined until a powerful sense of anticipation and craving emerges. Eventually, whether in a chilly MIT laboratory or your driveway, a habit is born.[4]

As you're reading this book, you'll hopefully become aware of many habits you may not have noticed before. If you embrace this awareness without judging yourself, seeking the cue and seeing more clearly the *almost* automatic nature of your response, your ability to instantaneously intercept that behavior will be greatly heightened. But do so compassionately, because being critical of yourself, inviting "a painful thought and feeling" will only impair your investigative skills, bringing on the very behaviors we're trying to avoid.

I urge you to expand your awareness, both of yourself and others, but to do so lovingly, noting what works, what needs tweaking, and looking forward to a plan. Perhaps you're still not buying the concept of becoming a "nondieter." "But I don't diet anymore," you may be thinking to yourself. "I eat whatever I please, but I'm still overweight and unhappy about it!"

There's another type of go-for-broke eating that's subtler, more pervasive in some circles yet equally damaging to one's health. I sometimes think of it as counterrestrictive chronic overeating, an insidious side effect of dieting and the dieting mentality. It differs from bingeing in that it's less extreme and obvious, but it can be just as serious, because the individual involved is frequently overweight, maybe even dangerously so, and has a sense of pseudofreedom from food restrictions and compulsive overeating. Let's look at an example of this syndrome, which can also be simply referred to as postdieting defiance. Although the anecdote has religious overtones (or irreligious, as it may be!), it's illustrative of the long-term effects of specific food restrictions.

I did my undergraduate training at a small university whose student population was predominantly Jewish. One day, I remember standing at the end of the cafeteria line with a Christian friend who said to me, "I can't believe the way people eat bacon at this college." She was commenting on a student who was heaping his plate with bacon, a sight I'd seen before and didn't question. As you may know, any meat derived from a pig is forbidden to those who follow the laws of kosher eating, as was probably practiced in a number of the households from which these students sprang. The fact that bacon was only an accompaniment to a main course and was usually eaten sparingly was news to me, given the gargantuan portions I'd often seen at that school.

This type of "Don't tell me not to!" eating is prevalent in our society and is a direct but frequently subconscious response to messages we receive about restricting our choice of foods. Acquiring an awareness of this tendency in oneself and in others is the first step toward change.

Here's another illustration. I'm an avid skier and years ago found myself sitting on a chair lift in Colorado with a gray-haired gentleman who disclosed that he was a cardiologist. As our conversation continued he asked about my work and specialties. When I mentioned compulsive overeating he immediately commented, "This should give you a chuckle. When I was back in the lodge a moment ago, I came upon a family I've worked with for years. They all have a family history that renders them prone to heart attacks in their forties and fifties, yet there they were, sitting around a large table eating breakfast and every one of them must have had a six-egg omelet. You should have seen their faces

when they saw me!" (Eggs seem no longer to be as dire a risk as formerly thought, but more on food choices in a later chapter.)

Counterrestrictive overeating can be chronic or occasional. Not long
ago I realized that I frequently felt uncomfortable on Saturday nights
after eating dinner out and even experienced heartburn and indigestion. Upon introspection I realized that, yes, I myself was suffering from
the syndrome, in which I was eating a number of heavy foods—although not necessarily consuming any one of them in great quantity—
merely because I was no longer a dieter and thought, "Darn it, yes I
can!" Admittedly, this resembles a postadolescent rebellion, in which a
rule is broken merely for the thrill of breaking it rather than for any real
pleasure in the activity.

Remember the pastry lady referred to earlier? We can imagine how
uncomfortably full she must have felt after finishing that platter. That's
not true freedom from restrictions. It's emotional overeating and could
be the beginning of a binge.

Yes, the bacon boys and the pastry lady share numerous characteristics, most notably the illusion that they're eating freely. Living now in
South Florida, I see many variations on these themes. It's most visible
at eateries known for rich foods in large portions (cheesecake, for example). Patrons stand in line for hours at certain venues, awaiting large,
heavy meals, only to emerge later wearing expressions indicating that
rather than feeling satisfied, they're merely stuffed and sad.

Dieting and counterrestrictive eating are mirror images of each other, both indicative of an unhealthy relationship with food. Dieters don't
feel free to eat; chronic overeaters aren't free to stop. The tragic result
of being trapped in one or both of these behaviors is that much of the
joy of food and life is lost.

Several years ago I worked with a single woman in her midtwenties
who taught elementary school and lived at home with her parents. A
pretty and intelligent young woman, Laura was also obese. Her inter-
nist, who was eager for health reasons that Laura lose weight, sent her
to me. Laura immediately told me that she'd been on every diet imagin-
able and that she didn't want to severely restrict her food choices again.

We eventually went out to eat a meal together and used the eating
techniques I'll later describe. Amazed at how soon she became full and
that she didn't need to finish at least half of what was on her plate, she
loved the experience. But returning to her familiar environment and

habits posed challenges. For example, her typical lunch was three cheeseburgers, which she ate while she was driving her car. When we discussed the option of her cutting that down to eating one cheeseburger while sitting in the restaurant, savoring it slowly, she became furious and temporarily suspended treatment.

Only sometime later was she willing to continue our work and consider consuming two cheeseburgers as she relaxed, listening to music in her parked vehicle. This was an interim step in cutting down her food intake further, expanding her eating awareness, and eventually exploring better choices.

Ask yourself the following questions and try to be as honest with yourself as you can. Do you find yourself frequently feeling uncomfortably full after meals, especially those eaten out? Do your clothes feel tight after you've eaten, especially after a meal not eaten at home? Do you often experience heartburn and other signs of indigestion? Do you frequently judge a restaurant by the heftiness of its portions?

If you've answered "yes" to even one of these questions, you may have at least a mild to moderate case of counterrestrictive overeating, a hindrance to you in feeling free to love your food. The techniques we'll discuss in chapter 5, about hands-on techniques, should prove helpful, along with other suggestions on maximizing satisfaction while savoring sensible portions.

If, on the other hand, you're consciously dieting, ask yourself now exactly how you feel about eating whatever you wish. Most likely it's still very scary to you. You might feel tempted to do so, but there's the sense that you're abandoning the dream of attaining the shape you desire. You may feel desperate for an immediate transformation so that anything less than a Spartan regime seems sinful. If you're desperate for immediate results, it's that attitude that will need to be reshaped before you can control your weight.

How do you feel about your body? Accepting yourself and your shape as you are is crucial if you aspire to change. If the very thought of your body as it currently looks and feels proves painful to you, then that, in itself, causes stress. As we have noted, that type of thinking and the painful feelings it produces are key factors in creating the need to compulsively overeat.

When I do seminars I'll frequently ask the audience, "Who here likes your body? Raise your hand." The response is usually paltry.

I'll then pose a series of questions. "Who here is relatively free of pain? Didn't most, if not all, of you walk into this room without assistance? Can you see me?" Little by little the audience realizes all the reasons they have to be grateful for their health and physical abilities. This is far different from our usual tendency, to some degree driven by the diet market, to berate our bodies and ourselves because we don't exactly meet some arbitrary standard of beauty. It's probable that your body is serving you well and possible that there are aspects of your appearance you actually like. What aspect of yourself do you visually enjoy? Your eyes? Your hair? The shape of your wrist? Your shoulders? Let yourself feel pride in any parts of your body that currently please you. In time you may be pleasantly surprised to find you possess other appealing physical characteristics, as well.

In her recent intimate and moving memoir, *Hunger*, Roxane Gay speaks up for those of us who feel that the way we look doesn't completely conform (and isn't that most of us?) to the ideal:

> It would be easy to pretend I am just fine with my body as it is. I wish I did not see my body as something for which I should apologize or provide explanation. I'm a feminist and I believe in doing away with the rigid beauty standards that force women to conform to unrealistic ideals. I believe we should have broader definitions of beauty that include diverse body types. I believe it is important for women to feel comfortable in their bodies, without wanting to change every single thing about their bodies to find that comfort. I (want to) believe my worth as a human being does not reside in my size or appearance. I know, having grown up in a culture that is generally toxic to women and constantly trying to discipline women's bodies, that it is important to resist unreasonable standards for how my body or any body should look. What I know and what I feel are two very different things.[5]

We can't help but cheer for the eloquent and intellectually enlightened woman who wrote these words. Her quest is laudable, but the challenges in today's society especially are daunting. Although Roxane Gay's intellectual evolution seems impressive, it sounds as if, not surprising in our current culture, she doesn't yet feel strong enough to lovingly embrace herself—both in body and mind.

Let's try our best to do this for ourselves. It's an important step in our efforts to move past emotional overeating. As for Ms. Gay, the self-awareness expressed in her writing is awesome. Let's hope it paves the way for future epiphanies—and that she shares them.

Does self-acceptance seem a strange stance at the start of this endeavor? At this point you may be expecting to be told about the importance of perfecting your body and that it's imperative that you immediately work to improve your appearance.

That's the catch-22 we face. To bring about positive behavioral change we need first to feel accepting toward ourselves. Reminding ourselves that we've done the best we could have done so far, given who we were then and what we knew until now, is powerfully therapeutic—even essential—to our efforts. But unless we meet an almost impossible cultural ideal, it's very difficult in our society to be self-accepting. People of all sizes and shapes, not only those who are overweight, receive negative feedback from others, especially those in marketing-oriented positions. Sadly, women can be the worst offenders toward each other.

Not long ago, I was working with Linda, a married woman in her forties who was a mother of two and a successful business consultant. To a large degree she'd resolved an eating disorder and had finally achieved a healthy, fit shape. She then decided to visit a local clothing store to buy some new outfits. It was a shop that catered to women who were middle-aged and older, though some of their clothes were trendy. After briefly perusing the stretch jeans, my client took a few off the rack and headed to the dressing room, pausing on the way to admire a black pantsuit. As she was doing so, the saleswoman approached and said, "You really should try *that* on. It hides everything!" My client, who had finally felt comfortable with her appearance and even at times proud of her body, subsequently backslid and it took us several sessions to undo the impact of that tactless but, unfortunately, not uncommon comment.

In a similar vein, I recently entered a local nutrition outlet to inquire about their diet pills. A teenage client was planning to try a certain brand and that caused me considerable concern. After I posed several questions about the side effects of the pill, the salesman launched into a high-powered sales pitch, pressuring me to purchase the product. Annoyed by this, I informed him I was inquiring only as a health professional, after which he asked, "What are you, a personal trainer?" To which I responded, "If that's your assumption how come you're trying to push weight loss pills on someone who doesn't need to lose weight?" For once, he was speechless.

It's hard to resist these market-driven messages that we can't be too slim too soon and that we dare not like our bodies as they are. Allow yourself to feel good about who you are and how you look right now. If you don't, your painful thoughts and feelings about yourself and your appearance will invade your life, making it difficult, if not impossible, to learn to eat in the moment, in a pleasure-oriented way.

Allow yourself to notice any negative thoughts you have about your body, the names you call yourself, or the criticisms you use. Rather than trying to immediately eradicate that behavior, simply become aware of it, shifting your attention when possible to more pleasant subjects, including aspects of yourself and your body for which you feel grateful. This will provide you some preliminary practice in the skills you'll learn in the chapters on stress and eating techniques.

The approach may still seem strange—especially as we start our work. Many of us believe that if we harbor any "imperfections" we need to whip ourselves into shape, a philosophy that's counterproductive when dealing with psychological change. Painful thoughts and feelings can contribute to a compulsion to escape into food by "stuffing" rather than savoring. And it's the latter—savoring—that you'll be learning to practice. Rather than radical changes in our thoughts or behavior, we'll be looking at how we can tweak our habitual styles of thinking, feeling, and behaving, preserving what's useful and unique about ourselves while improving what we need to change.

So allow yourself to feel good about who you are and how you look right now. Begin by starting to honor yourself and your wishes. You might, for example, choose to buy yourself some attractive clothing that looks great on you exactly as you are. Treat yourself to some up-to-date accessories, or that perfume or cologne you haven't indulged in for years.

During the day occasionally ask yourself whether you're hungry and what exactly it is you crave. Choose to eat only what pleases you. At first you may overeat some foods you crave most, especially if you've been consciously restricting them. Sit down and give whatever you eat your total attention. If you long for a chocolate bar, for example, try to buy just one at a time. But really taste it. You can always have another one tomorrow if you choose. There's no need to eat one and feel guilty, eat two and feel worse, and then eat a third in a desperate attempt to drown the resultant guilt. Take note of what you like and even dislike about the treat you've decided to try. This will be an important introduction to eating mindfully—truly being in the moment as you eat.

When I was a compulsive eater I'd often long for chocolate and would occasionally succumb to what I considered my "naughty" impulses and buy an oversize Hershey bar. Sometimes I'd eat this on the way home from work as I walked the streets of Manhattan's Upper East Side, barely tasting it as I browsed in store windows, dodged taxis, and dealt with the crowds and the noise. This loosening of self-restraint would evoke a sense of guilt and self-loathing that would sometimes balloon into a full-blown binge. After I'd developed a slightly better handle on this behavior, I'd sometimes buy the bar, break it in half, and carefully place the remaining portion, wrapped, upon the nearest waste receptacle for a homeless person to find.

I still love chocolate and eat it whenever I wish. How do I currently indulge? A favorite pleasure is to stop at a Godiva Chocolatier, located in a local, elegant, and comfy mall. I'll usually buy one "opened oyster," their best-selling confection, a wonderful mélange of milk chocolate and smooth, creamy hazelnut praline. First, I'll sit comfortably in one of the cozy couches, looking forward to slowly savoring small bites of the one small piece of chocolate I've purchased. Then I'll lean back, feasting on the sight, scent, taste, and texture of this unique confection as I pleasurably gaze at people passing by. While I savor the smooth texture and sumptuous milky taste, my thoughts may wander to my late, beloved mother, who also adored this edible delight. This in turn recalls soothing reminiscences of watching her savor the same treat. Because my enjoyment of the experience is so fulfilling, it isn't something I need to do often. And best of all, I know I can evoke the calming recollections at will, with or without consuming the candy.

Are there items that evoke similarly soothing associations for you and that you can also savor? Try to do so, whether at a mall, during a meal, or whenever. But concentrate on really being there as you do. Make sure you get the greatest possible pleasure from any food you love.

If you're presently dieting, this may seem scary. But let me assure you that as we move on not only will we be looking at how you can eat whatever you like; we'll be placing equal emphasis on how you can tune in to fullness and satisfaction and then *stop*.

Now that you're periodically asking yourself what might please your palate, it's time to ask yourself another, equally if not more important, question. What would bring joy in other ways to your day? Perhaps there are activities or hobbies that you've put on hold or have never dared to try. Even if your routine is fairly regimented, there are opportunities to add some joy if you're creative. Try doing something at work in a slightly different way. During your lunchtime try taking a walk down a beckoning but formerly unexplored path. If you have children, or pets, try a new activity with them. Start to think about opening yourself up to new opportunities to live your life more fully.

Focusing solely on controlling our eating is self-defeating. We've already explored some reasons for this and have seen how broken restrictions can result in bingeing. But there's another important way in which dieting can destroy our love of food and life. The dieter, in a desperate attempt to lose weight, endeavors to eat less and not dwell on food. But resolving *not* to think about anything is impossible. There's a classic demonstration often done in psychotherapy groups or classes in which the therapist asks everyone in the room not to think about a pink elephant. Can you guess the results? Try to do it. He's adorable, isn't he? It's impossible—unless you eventually allow yourself to think of something else.

Julia Cameron, whose inspirational work *The Artist's Way* helped give me the courage to write this book, offers many wonderful suggestions for saying yes to yourself and putting pleasure into your life. She encourages her readers to ignore all those who doubt their abilities and to go ahead and do whatever they want to do, whether the results are perfect or not.

The most frequent answer I get when I question clients about why they want to lose weight is "I want to be happy." When I was in college I had a beautiful poster that I placed on the wall in my dormitory room. It had flowers and butterflies on it and the saying below them read: "Happiness is like a butterfly. If you chase it, it will fly away. But when you busy yourself with other things, it will come and gently perch upon your shoulder."

Ask yourself what might bring new joy and comfort into your life. If you can't immediately make it happen, ask yourself how you'd know that you were moving in that direction. Then do whatever you need to do to take that first, then second, then third step along the way. Each step might take only five minutes or less. It could be Googling a Meet-up group, or phoning an adult education center in your area. If starting seems scary, then ask yourself, "What would I do *if* I were planning to begin that activity?" Then take the steps and see how you feel as you go along.

One of the benefits of attending events lies in the opportunity to ask people about all the things they do to keep active and involved. "What other things do you do for fun?" may open up new ideas about pleasurable pastimes.

If you don't immediately feel interested in your new activity, remember that, frequently, involvement precedes interest. It may take a while for your new involvement to become an interest and for that interest to become a passion. One of those passions, however, might even eventually develop into a lifelong dream. Dare to find a dream and follow it. If you aren't sure what that dream might be, don't despair. Just allow yourself to start to think about what would make you feel more alive. Open yourself up, right now, to all the possibilities for pleasurable productivity and creativity in your life.

Find new ways to enjoy life more each day. Ask yourself what or who has been preventing you from taking piano lessons, adopting a pet (adult dogs, who abound in shelters, need relatively little care), learning a foreign language, taking that tango class, joining that foreign affairs club, reading a classic with your child, or even going for that degree you've always coveted.

Whatever you decide to do needn't be time-consuming nor expensive. What's important is that you become aware of adopting a new outlook in which you tell yourself that you deserve to enjoy every day of your life. Start using some of your free moments to think creatively about how to do this.

It's now time to look at another way of expanding your awareness and improving your life, a very intimate way of acknowledging and honoring your thoughts, feelings, sensations, and ultimately yourself. It's the process of journaling. I recommend setting up a time each day to write a few pages—a blog from you to you. Think of this as a very important time, an unbreakable "date" with yourself. Use whatever time it takes to fill some pages with a conversation with yourself. Write about whatever you choose—your thoughts, your feelings, your hopes, your dreams (those while you're awake or asleep).

If you do remember your dreams, they can be a wonderful key to opening doors of self-awareness that would otherwise be closed. Tune in to the feelings in your dream—joy, sadness, anger, and anxiety. They're clues to underlying emotions you may be experiencing but not acknowledging during your day. Next, notice what's happening in the dream. Is it a metaphor in any way for something meaningful happening in your life? Examining our dreams can be a positive step toward growth and change.

Write about any experiences that catch your attention, whether they bring you joy, pain, or a combination of both. Share with yourself as you would with a kindly, attentive friend. You might choose to write down your feelings about starting this work.

One client, Beth, was beginning her sessions with me when she had the following dream. She was going to visit her grandmother, who, in actuality was deceased, but in the dream was very ill. Although she expected to see her grandmother in a coma when she approached, Beth noted that the old woman's eyes were open and that she was looking at her clearly.

When we looked at the dream together Beth realized that she had felt happiness and relief that her grandmother was alive and could see her, "that her eyes were open." Yet when I asked her about her waking associations to her grandmother, she said that her grandmother had been a very angry, unhappy woman. The dream indicated a burgeoning self-awareness on Beth's part, which pleased her, but it also pointed the way to emotional realities she'd have to work on if she was to conquer her overeating. Once her eyes were opened to her sadness and her anger, Beth could start to console herself and heal. But she'd have to "look it in the face" before she could make peace with these emotions and with herself.

Let your thoughts, feelings, and imagination flow freely. Try not to censor anything. Accept your myriad emotions with openness and curiosity, rather than adopting a rigid judgmental stance. That's the way you'll learn and grow most rapidly.

Saying no to dieting really means saying yes to pleasure, to accepting yourself, your body, thoughts, and feelings. It means allowing an expanded awareness of your wishes and your world. It means no longer denying yourself the right to do what you've always dreamed of doing. If you can't immediately conjure a passion you'd potentially like to pursue, just open yourself up to the possibility that your dream is there, waiting for you to find it, if you allow yourself to embrace it. That's exciting, isn't it?

For me, the writing of this book was the realization of a dream—the dream to help more people than I'd previously imagined to more fully enjoy their food and their lives. The writing of this book has been a pleasurable process, during which I've often almost forgotten where I was, who I was, and even, believe it or not, when I was to eat my next meal. There may well be at least one book in you as well, but whatever your choice of goal, or goals, make it something meaningful. It could have to do with those you love—being a better father, or husband, or sister, or wife. Perhaps it has to do with your role as a caring and loving friend. It may have to do with making your daily work more enjoyable or easier for yourself, your colleagues, or staff, or with doing your work in a more creative and exciting way. It may have to do with taking a hobby to the next level—selling your paintings, or sculpture, or even teaching your talent to a group. Make it something that helps you to get out of bed with a smile, excited because it's another day in which you dare to pursue your dream.

Now you're ready for the first letter of your first mnemonic device. It's the beginning of the one-minute monitor, a word you remember each day to remind yourself to take part in the behavioral tweaks advised in this book. It's the first letter of the word **SELF**—an **S**. Remember it by asking yourself each day if you're doing what's best for your "self."

What does the **S** stand for? It stands for the subject of the next chapter—**S**tress. Managing stress on your own without food—learning to self-soothe—is central to letting go of emotional overeating.

We've covered a lot and you may want to give it all some thought. When you're ready, let's move forward.

3

POINT #1: STRESS—LEARN FROM IT TO LESSEN IT

"Stop the Stress!"—"Give Holiday Stress the Boot"—"50 Ways to Banish Stress"

You may see these and similar headlines while you're checking out at the supermarket, surfing the net, or as intros to TV segments. But while these promises are appealing, it's important to remember that true stress management isn't about abolishing stress. It's about facing—even embracing—all we experience, enabling us to learn and grow.

We live in a society where savoring solitude—actually enjoying our emotions and ourselves rather than merely tolerating time alone—is considered controversial. We're tuned in to outside stimuli constantly, via cell phones, the internet, television, or several technologies at once. But tuning out distractions and tuning in to our thoughts and feelings, even the unpleasant ones, can yield essential information, not just about what we're experiencing, but, most important, about how we characteristically treat ourselves.

"How well do I treat myself?" "Do I really care for myself in a loving and respectful way?" "When the chips are down, am I supportive of my efforts whether they succeed or not?" These may be questions you rarely ask yourself, especially during tense times. Unfortunately, during times of stress, many of us, especially those with a tendency to compulsively overeat, aren't able to pause and pose these crucial questions. We feel painfully alone and isolated, not only from others, but, worst of all, from ourselves.

In working with the bereaved at hospitals, at Cancer Care, and in my practice, it's not been uncommon to hear clients say, "I lost my parents. I've lost my husband. I have *nobody*." If you ever feel that way, remember something crucial: You are not alone. You have someone very special—*yourself*.

Sadly, many of us often forget to take good care of the one person who's always present in our lives. Often unaware of it, we neglect, disparage, and disrespect ourselves, especially during difficult times.

How do we develop these habits? Why isn't it natural for many of us to treat ourselves in a kindly, nurturing way, especially when life deals a tough blow? One of the most powerful ways we learn how to treat ourselves emanates from the way our early caregivers treated not only us, but themselves, as well. The way they lived their lives and handled or mishandled stress sent powerful messages, not only in terms of what they said, but also by what they did.

While none of us have had perfect childhoods, the type of nurturing we received and the way our parents treated themselves sent strong messages. If you're currently going through a difficult time, think about your parents and how they'd react, or would have reacted, to your situation. If you didn't know one or both of your parents, consider your caregiver's responses and how that felt for you. If you didn't feel supported in times of emotional pain, if you didn't feel nurtured and loved whether you succeeded or failed, then I feel for you. You've experienced a very real emotional loss.

As Alice Miller states in *Prisoners of Childhood*, "That greatest of all narcissistic wounds, not to have been loved just as one truly was, cannot be healed without the work of mourning."[1] Most of us have been wounded in some way. Yet many of us fail to acknowledge that we experienced this trauma. Only by acknowledging that loss, working through the feelings, and showing compassion to ourselves as we were, and as we are now, can we heal.

Try this brief exercise. Take yourself back to your childhood and a room in the home of your family of origin. Feel the feelings that being in that room elicited. Was it light, dark, happy, sad, open, closed to the world, safe and secure, or somehow dangerous? Let the feelings flow. Bring in significant family members. What were (or are) their characteristic expressions? Cheerful? Worried? Angry? Depressed? Sit there for a moment. Is this painful? If so, how? Remember what it was like for you when you felt stressed at that time. Picture a time when you felt an unfulfilled desire or an emotional need. What kind of responses did you get? Were they helpful or not? If not, what would you have wished that your parents or caregivers would have said or done? If loving people weren't present, let yourself feel the sadness, the sense of loss, even abandonment. Feel for the child within you, then and now, who sometimes feels uncomfortably alone.

Play around with this scenario, allowing yourself to change whatever you'd like, not just facial expressions, verbal and nonverbal responses, but even details of the setting, such as opening windows and letting in more sunlight, if that would bring you joy. Try this exercise using different rooms—places in which your family may have slept, played, or ate. Each of these scenarios will bring you important remembrances of how you felt then and how you would have liked to have felt. This can be a very powerful exercise. The beauty of it lies in that you're feeling for yourself and your former losses, but you are also allowing yourself—the adult you are today—to take control.

Leah, a middle-aged married woman with three teenagers, struggled with bouts of depression as well as compulsive overeating. When she "felt" back into her childhood she pictured herself eating dinner alone in a dark gloomy dining room. Her parents, who cooked for a catering firm, were often working events at night. When they were home, the situation wasn't much better. Both of her parents had been Holocaust survivors. Leah's mother would often sit alone in a room, sometimes with the lights out, staring into space. Leah, the child, felt guilt about not being able to heal her mother's pain, thinking (as children often do) that she should have had the ability to "magically" control her world. In spite of Leah's lack of nurturing, she became a loving mother, vowing to give her children what she had not received. The emotional needs she did abandon, however, were her own.

Doing this exercise may cause us to remember how helpless we felt during our childhood—our painful awareness of our inability to change our environment and those around us in a way that would afford us comfort. One key aspect of food's allure is its ready availability as a mood modifier—albeit a momentary one. Recall again the definition given earlier of emotional overeating—*Emotional overeating can be defined as eating neither for enjoyment nor for the satisfaction of hunger, but in a desperate attempt to distract oneself from painful thoughts and feelings*. Numbing out, stuffing down feelings, closet eating often begin in our earliest home, where we were powerless to make more meaningful and permanent changes.

If doing this kind of work leaves you angry, allow yourself to experience that emotion. This may feel uncomfortable, whether the anger is new or whether you've owned it for a while. If you believe that it's wrong to feel anger toward parents, spouses, or children, or if you fault yourself for feeling hate toward those you love, you'll be prone to try to escape a very uncomfortable feeling. And what may be your substance of choice?

Cookies, anyone? And not just a few!

It's important to accept that we all feel ambivalence toward people in our lives, even toward ourselves. It's normal and okay. Accepting the wide range of feelings we may have toward loved ones, friends, jobs, homes, organizations, any of the important persons or aspects of our life, can be liberating.

Why do so many of us attempt to ignore, rather than honor, our inner lives? The answer lies in part in the way we were treated as children and the role models we saw. But another part of the answer lies in the success-oriented, in some ways superficial, society in which we live. It's hard not to feel uncomfortable if we acknowledge, even to ourselves, that we're upset.

Imagine your reaction if an acquaintance says, "Are you okay? You seem stressed." Or if he or she comments, "Is anything the matter? You look depressed." Your knee-jerk reaction might be, "No, I'm fine. Everything's okay." Inside, however, you know that it's not. Because that distress has been noticed, you may feel even more disconcerted, embarrassed, and vulnerable. "Someone has noticed I'm out of control. How did I let that happen?"

But the beauty of experiencing this *awareness*—an important word throughout our work—is that only by doing so can you regain real control of your emotions and your life.

As an analogy, remember how you felt when you were a child and fell and bruised your knee? You experienced the pain, looked to see if a bruise existed, and then probably cried aloud, running to seek a parent or caretaker for relief and comfort. As adults, however, we often ignore emotional pain or try to tell ourselves that it doesn't exist. "I'm just irritable today," we may say to ourselves, or "It's just that my husband/

sister/best friend/mother-in-law really ticked me off!" Or, "Nothing's going right for me today, so what's the point in dwelling on it?"

Believing that it's futile to confront emotional pain prevents us from acknowledging, understanding, and overcoming it. This reminds me of a phenomenon often faced by skiers—the mound-shaped bumps on a slope called moguls, which some skiers see as hurdles and try to avoid. However, by skiing toward a mogul, bending your knees, and turning on top, the mogul serves to unweight you, allowing you to pivot almost effortlessly—thereby making the turn easier.

Likewise, there's much to be learned from emotional pain that frees you, both emotionally and physically, if you're brave enough to face it and to learn from the experience. "But I often don't understand what's happening" you may say. "All I know is that I'm feeling lousy, upset, unmotivated. . . ." In that case, what's the point of delving further and exploring our emotional pain?

The truth is that understanding our stress—using it before we can lose it—yields real rewards in making our lives better. The other option, attempting to escape our emotions by "stuffing" them down with food, is both uninformative and fattening! So the next time you're feeling irritated, upset, slightly blue, or anxious, try using this new approach. Your goal is to get to the point where you can say to yourself, "Hello stress. What are you trying to tell me? What are you trying to teach me so that I can comfort myself and learn to gain control?"

While in the throes of excessive stress, however, it's almost impossible to be objective about what's happening. So I'm going to provide a set of strategies I'll refer to as the **ABCD**s of stress management. As you may have already guessed, the **A** is for **A**wareness, the crucial first step in taking charge of our emotional state.

How do we sense that we're experiencing excessive stress? There are many discernable signs, including rapid heartbeat, shallow breathing, muscular tension, "edginess" or a heightened startle response, an inability to concentrate, and irritability. In addition, you may have other specific symptoms that are characteristic of your personal response to tension, such as headaches, back pain, gastrointestinal ailments, facial twitches, or some combination of the above.

Certain behaviors may also clue you in that you're emotionally distressed on a less conscious level. It's helpful to learn to identify your own unique style, and to do so without self-recrimination. Other stress-related behaviors may include snapping at coworkers, your partner, or your children; making mistakes at work or at home; dropping things and other accidental behaviors; and, for compulsive overeaters, either bingeing or making preparations to eat excessively. Drifting toward the fridge and starting to eat in a mindless manner without hunger can be a crucial clue that something is emotionally amiss. This may be due to a stress-related distraction that's causing you to revert from your healthy new habits—like the eating techniques we'll learn later. Try to detect these indicators of distress so that learning opportunities aren't lost.

When you spot these behaviors and the heightened stress level they denote, avoid making painful judgments. Your ultimate goal may be to lessen or eradicate these behaviors, but to do so you'll have to first observe and understand them. Don't expect to be able to do this immediately. If you're feeling irritable, upset, or pained, that's probably the worst time to try to analyze and assess your emotional situation.

Which leads us to the next step—step **B**, for Taking a **B**reak. It's often necessary to take a break before we can analyze what's occurring within us and take charge of our emotions and reactions. Before we can take charge, we must relax and regroup.

So do whatever you need to do to put a "pause" on your emotional pain. Do something that will temporarily relax and distract you, in a healthy, productive way. Chat with a supportive friend, exercise, take deep breaths or stretch, take a walk around the block, or engage in a favorite hobby. Your goal is to gain some emotional distance from the internal or external source of your distress so that you'll be able to approach your situation more objectively.

Some of my personal favorite breaks include calling good friends, playing the piano, walking, and tossing a ball to Red, our redbone hound—a former pound pup. Develop your own repertoire of non-food-related breaks so that you have a choice of behaviors readily available wherever you may be.

When you feel you've achieved a little distance from your distress you're ready for step three, **C**, which involves Noticing the **C**hange you're experiencing. This way you can approach the "crisis" in the spirit of the Chinese, who write the word utilizing symbols for two concepts—danger and opportunity.

Let's begin this step with a brief definition of stress, from the classic work by Hans Selye, *The Stress of Life*:

> Stress is the non-specific response of the body to any demand, whether it is caused by or results in, pleasant or unpleasant conditions. Good or bad, pleasant or unpleasant are already specific features of our response to a demand, just as cold or heat are specific variants of temperature changes. Stress, as such, just as temperature as such, is all-inclusive, embodying both the positive and negative aspects of these concepts. We must, however, differentiate within the general concept of stress between the unpleasant or harmful variety, called "distress" (from the Latin dis = bad, as in dissonance, disagreement) and "eustress" (from the Greek eu = good, as in euphonia, euphoria). During both eustress and distress the body undergoes virtually the same nonspecific responses to the various positive or negative stimuli acting upon it. However, the fact that eustress causes much less damage than distress graphically demonstrates that it is *"how you take it"* that determines, ultimately, whether you can adapt successfully to change.[2]

Notice the final sentence of Selye's analysis here. Different people may respond to the same external event in different ways, or may respond differently to the same event at different times; this is a very important concept and one we'll revisit.

Frequently, when I see a new client, especially someone who states they are struggling with stress, a mutual exploration of the client's life reveals telltale signs of change. For example, the client's supervisor at work may have been replaced, a relative with whom the client has a conflicted relationship has just moved close by, or a milestone birthday is approaching.

In the latter case it's often helpful to explore the significance of that year. Was there a "to-do list" that was supposed to be checked off by that age? Understanding their expectations of their world and themselves often affords important answers.

What's so stressful about change? While certain situations may be inherently painful—the loss of a family member, getting fired, experiencing a serious illness, or divorce—there are other types of change that many of us assume will be purely pleasurable: "the eustress" to which Selye referred.

Pleasurable changes may include vacations, an engagement, the holiday season, or awards for exceptional achievement. However, what often comes with these occasions can be "clusters of change," which, while individually might not be significant, taken together can be quite challenging. Vacations may bring differences in climate, language, eating patterns and types of food available, activity levels, altitude, types of companionship, and, of course, packing.

With holiday season comes the expectation of happy celebrations, along with more frequent family get-togethers (sometimes with people we find difficult), the pressure of purchasing gifts, and perhaps hosting responsibilities. The expectation (engendered to a great extent by advertising) that the holidays feature multiple generations of smiling, happy, healthy family members, every couple accompanied by 2.3 children, serenely spending time together, is one of the reasons that depression has been palpable at any health care organization I've worked at from November through New Year's.

Many types of change are stressful because they involve adjustments not only to our behavior, but to our self-concept as well—often in ways that are new and unexpected. Take, for example, the situation of a person who's just won a long-sought-after promotion. At first there's a great deal of excitement (again, what Selye terms eustress) related to the validation one feels, the higher salary, larger office, and so on. But then self-doubt may settle in as the newly promoted employee begins to wonder if he or she will be able to perform the new job-related tasks. Formerly friendly colleagues may now harbor envy and resentment. There may be frustration at the long hours and lack of cooperation from staff or peers. The new position may come with a new supervisor, who may or may not be as supportive as the last one.

When faced with change, we must adjust our expectations—not only of our world but also of ourselves. The new reality may not live up to our former fantasies. If we expect perfection in ourselves or in our lives, we're especially prone to feel tension, anxiety, and depression. Any seasoned therapist can tell you that when a client raves about a perfect new mate, new job, or new home, depression may be arriving soon, as well.

This takes us back to Selye's words about the cause of stress, specifically, that it's not just the external events, but "how you take it." This concept is the cornerstone of one of the most exciting, effective, and practical developments in psychotherapy today—cognitive behavioral therapy (CBT). And the best thing about CBT is that it's easy to understand and learn, so that you can use it to subdue stress, nurture yourself, and become more self-soothing.

The basic myth that CBT challenges is the belief that you're feeling stress solely because of external circumstances, when, to a great extent, your feelings are actually caused by your *thoughts*. The chain of events set in motion can be seen as a spiral, swirling upward or downward, as illustrated in the accompanying figures. When we notice the phenomenon that's taking place—that our *thoughts* are causing our *feelings* that are causing our choice of behavior—we can then take control and create an upward, more positive progression.

Many of us think that external events cause us to have certain feelings, which then create our moods, determine our behavior, leading us uncontrollably onward, often on a downward, unproductive course. Examine figure 3.1 as an example of this "pre-CBT" type of paradigm, noting how irrevocably out of control it looks and feels.

If you choose, plug in an event that recently caused you anguish. Taking the time to personalize these concepts will help to make them more memorable, as well. Ask yourself what happened, how you felt and acted, and whether that behavior perpetuated itself in a manner that was helpful or harmful. Do not judge. Just notice.

You may choose to write down the external event that preceded the pain (here referred to as the Stressor), and then the feeling or mood, as well as the behavior that followed. Did the incident result in a situation in which you felt regrettably out of control?

Now take a look at figure 3.2. What do you observe here that's different? First of all, look at the upper-left portion of the diagram. Whereas before we had the term *Stressor*, we now have *Potential Stressor* instead. Why is that? To a great extent the term *stressor* is subjective. Certain situations that are stressful to you may not be stressful to me. Conversely, I may find some situations stressful that you may consider a breeze. For example, I wouldn't mind skiing down a fairly steep slope, but put me in a pool with water that's over my head and I'm not happy. Either or both of those situations might seem really easy to you.

Another question I often ask clients is this: "Would you find the thought of it raining tomorrow stressful?" Usually the answer is no (although occasionally I'll get a "Not another bad hair day!" response). Then I'll ask, "But what if you'd planned an outdoor wedding, engagement, or birthday party?" Then I'll usually get a "Yes, that'd be scary"

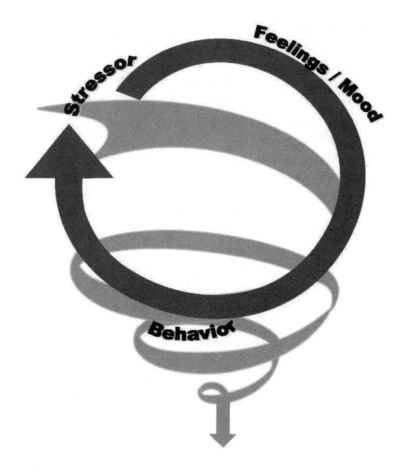

Figure 3.1.   Pre–Cognitive Behavioral Therapy Stress Model

answer. And then I'll ask, "But what if you'd planned for contingencies with a tent, or if the bride-to-be loved artsy, sun-peeping-through-the-clouds photos? And so on." Again, the response will change.

Our degree of stress varies greatly according to our attitude toward events as well as their circumstances. But the greatest component of our attitude is the second thing that's different in figure 3.2. Look again and what do you see? It's the addition of another concept—that of our *thoughts*. And that's because it's our thoughts that create our feelings, which in turn create our moods and lead to our behavior. This cycle can move, sadly, in a spiral leading downward, unproductively, as seen in figure 3.1. Or, as in figure 3.2, the cycle may evolve upward, toward

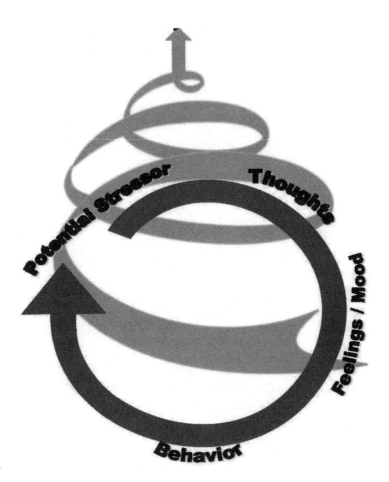

Figure 3.2. Cognitive Behavioral Therapy Stress Model

resolution and control—to the greatest extent possible given the situation.

What is it that enables us to take back control?

Yes, it's our *thoughts*. That's because one of the key concepts of CBT is that it's not just the situation itself that can cause our stress. Our characteristic patterns of thought can not only add to the stress of a situation but even create it.

So how can we take back control? Again, we return to that key word *awareness*. By becoming *aware* of the thoughts we're experiencing— our personal style of speaking to ourselves—we're able to observe if these thoughts are helping us by creating comfort or, unfortunately, habitually hurting us by producing pain.

If you find that you're experiencing thoughts that not only add to your stress but create it, don't despair, and by all means don't feel disappointed in yourself. I've given seminars on this subject to law firm associates, an emergency medicine department in a metropolitan hospital, large groups of young moms, and so forth, and, invariably, when I speak of thoughts that cause pain, every head in the room nods in recognition!

Let's look at some examples of what I call *pain-producing thoughts*, which most of us experience at times. The first one we'll examine was referred to by Karen Horney, one of the first eminent female psychoanalysts, as "the tyranny of the shoulds"[3] and is often a sign of perfectionism. Reconsidering the example used above of the promotion, we can imagine the employee thinking that others "should" be less resentful and more cooperative or that the new responsibilities of the position "should" be less challenging. It's obvious that this type of blame and this sense of unfairness can prevent us from adapting and evolving in a new scenario.

Birthday-related depression is another example that may also be related to the tyrannical "shoulds." It's not unusual for clients to feel sad as they approach "a big one" and have an unrealistic expectation of where their lives "should" be at a certain age, causing a sense of failure or self-recrimination when these objectives haven't been achieved. "I should be married, have children, own a successful business. . . ." These are some of the goals that may be linked to specific ages in an individual's mind. It's far more compassionate to remind ourselves that people and life aren't always perfect, and that learning and growing and doing our best is more important than whether we arrive where we've expected to at the exact moment predicted.

Here's a more personal example of the tyranny of the shoulds, which relates to my own experience with this chapter. Writing this was very difficult for me at first, and for a while I procrastinated, even though I'm a seasoned psychotherapist who has led stress management and time management seminars for a wide range of audiences. Nevertheless, this was the hardest chapter to write. Why? Because I felt that, given my profession and experience, this "should" be the perfect, ultimate, definitive, all-inclusive, seminal work on the subject of stress—

and all in thirty pages or less! It was only upon uncovering this pain-producing thought that I was able to be aware of these self-defeating and unrealistic expectations and perceive the immense pressure I was placing on myself. Only then could I resume writing, knowing that while this chapter can, if necessary, be revised, it may never—like so much in life that's real—be perfect.

Closely related to the tyranny of the shoulds is another potentially pain-producing thought pattern, in which we see our lives and ourselves as either totally good or totally bad, without shades of gray in between. Examples of these thoughts are "I never do anything right," "My husband never helps me," or "My mother always criticizes me." Words like *always* and *never* are tip-offs that we're engaging in this pessimistic thought pattern, thereby blinding ourselves to a more positive interpretation of events. One of the many downsides of thinking this way is that we sabotage our strengths and become depressed and demoralized. This saps our confidence to learn from mistakes and move forward. In addition, we may then start to speak this way as well, lessening our chance of gaining understanding and cooperation from others. All in all it's a dangerous downward spiral.

Another style of pain-producing thought that can cause us a great deal of trouble is name-calling—referring to ourselves or others in terms that are negative. Examples include, "I'm fat"; "He's a jerk"; "My boss is a bitch." Referring to yourself as "fat" may well be a way of expressing anger about some perceived personal imperfection. Use your evolving self-awareness to notice that you have more of a tendency to do that when you're going through difficult changes in your life, regardless of your weight.

Celine, a beautiful, intelligent brunette in her twenties, referred to herself as "fat" at the beginning of a session. Upon exploration it became apparent that after she had quit her evening job she had been spending more time socializing in bars, often with a beautiful blond friend who'd been attracting more attention than Celine. Rather than analyze her situation—including the fact that bars might not be her best milieu for spending time or meeting men—Celine referred to herself as "fat." This enabled her to avoid important information, including a need for change. Not surprisingly, the painful self-accusations also served as an impetus for eating binges. Only after she examined her habitual pain-producing thoughts and the way this distracted her from seeking new solutions was she able to explore new ways of meeting men and move on toward meeting a future mate.

Feeling incriminated is another common pain-producing thought process. Sometimes we assume that a person or persons are treating us unfairly because of something specific about ourselves. While sometimes this may be so, and analyzing our behavior or others' prejudices may be in order, if we often feel we're being personally targeted, we may cause ourselves unnecessary pain.

One example that comes to mind is Gemma, a lovely, bright young woman who was interested in joining a women's group I was leading, but she asked me in advance not to call on her to speak unless she volunteered. She confessed that she felt very frightened in groups and wanted to have the opportunity to volunteer to speak only when she knew she felt ready. Several times during the group I asked for comments from the people present and occasionally, noting nonverbal reactions, requested feedback from members by name. Adhering to her request, however, I didn't summon Gemma. The following week she didn't show up for the meeting. When I inquired about her absence she told me that it was because I'd rejected her in the group. She felt I'd done so because she was "short" and that people often overlooked her for that reason! We discussed this at length to help her understand that it wasn't her height, but her specific request, born of her poor self-image, that explained her "exclusion."

Another painful thought pattern, which tends to produce anxiety, a frequent correlate of depression, is cataclysmic predictions. If you often fear the future, imagine the worst, expect the sky to be falling, and similarly "terrible-ize," you know all too well how uncomfortable these feelings can be. Perhaps in the past you experienced a great deal of hardship or lived with an adult who held a similar philosophy of gloom and doom. Recognizing this habit is the crucial first step toward regaining control and learning to recapture the joy in life.

What's the purpose of tuning in to these "pain-producers"? How does a pain-producer differ from less toxic thoughts? One way I find helpful to spot this type of thinking is by using a metaphor. Picture your mood as if it were the sky above you. If you see a dark cloud in a distant corner of the horizon, you're probably not in the throes of a pain-producing thought. However, if you sense a huge black cloud following you everywhere, all the time, covering your entire sky, that type of thinking indicates a painful pattern.

In other words, if the nature of your thought is

- **p**ermanent,
- **a**ll-encompassing,
- **i**ncriminating, and
- **n**egative,

it's probably a **pain**-producer!

Since two key symptoms of depression are hopelessness and helplessness, it is easy to see how the habit of holding pain-producing thought patterns produces depression. The beauty of catching yourself at these patterns is that once they are recognized, they can be changed, as we'll explore in step **D** in the **ABCD**s of stress management. For now, I'd like you to become more skillful, a detective of sorts, at spotting the clues that you're engaging in this hurtful habit. One clue that a thought is a pain-producer is that it reverberates repeatedly and is reminiscent of words your parents used when they were negative, unkind, or resigned.

One client, an intelligent, creative, middle-aged man, was underemployed and neglecting some admirable skills. He repeatedly voiced the question "What's the use?," reminiscent of his former absentee father who had been a substance abuser. Another client, who could not commit to meaningful relationships because of low self-esteem, often used the phrase "That's just my luck," reminiscent of a father who had been a compulsive gambler and had abandoned his wife and three sons for another woman. A young female client, prone to bingeing whenever she failed at any minor task, would repeatedly say to me and to herself, "Everything I do is wrong!" She was repeating the words of her mother, who struggled with ongoing severe depression throughout the client's childhood and adolescence.

Notice how you speak to yourself when you're alone. How do you treat yourself as you review the events of your day or your life? Observing your inner monologue will provide important clues as to how you treat yourself. The beauty of bringing this into awareness is that by doing so we can change the script, ease the pain, and compassionately take charge of our lives.

You may now be wondering whether we're ignoring the reality that certain circumstances are, in and of themselves, inherently painful. Certainly, many stressors like a loved one's death, divorce, severe illness, or losing a job would be difficult for anyone. But what's doubly tragic is that many of us unwittingly cause ourselves additional pain during troubled times.

How is this so? Sadly, in my many years at medical and psychiatric settings, including seven years at Cancer Care, Inc., I have often seen people engage in patterns of thought that add to rather than detract from their distress. Far too frequently we judge ourselves harshly for our actions or reactions during a time of trouble or loss.

The first type of pain-producing thought I encountered frequently at Cancer Care and at other medical settings was diminished self-esteem due to the advent of the illness or loss. Patients and family members alike often plagued themselves with thoughts like "Why did this happen to me? Why do I deserve this?" Sadly, the way some of us interpret our Judeo-Christian heritage leads to the feeling that if we are "blessed" with good health or good fortune we may therefore be "cursed" with the reverse. As Robert Chernin Cantor states in his brilliant book *And a Time to Live*, during a medical crisis there is often a disturbing confrontation with "the shadow self."[4] This is Jung's term for a negative self-image that can be elicited by any experience that causes us to question our sense of being always and unrealistically good, right, dependable, strong, or whatever other quality upon which we had hitherto based our sense of self-esteem. Having worked with thousands of people who were coping with the impact of medical, psychiatric, and other crises, I can attest that this syndrome is almost universal.

A second way in which people add to their pain during an already tough time has been referred to as "the if-only syndrome" by Ann Kliman in her wisdom-filled work *Crisis: Psychological First Aid for Recovery and Growth*.[5] This refers to the excruciating pain of self-recrimination after a loss (especially, but not exclusively, a sudden one), a disappointment, or whatever may be viewed as a costly mistake. This is often associated with a mental replay of the events leading up to the traumatic occurrence, with the fantasy that the change of one link in the chain of events would bring about a different, more desirable outcome. According to Kliman,

Magical thinking is not only indulged in by children, it is an adjustment reaction for most severely stressed adults. How often have you heard someone impose guilt on himself, say following an auto accident: "If only I hadn't sent her on that errand!"; or, following an infant's fall: "If only I hadn't been taking a shower!" If only, if only—as if we had the omnipotence to control life and death, or the omniscience to read the future.[6]

As Colin Parkes wrote in *Bereavement*, "The tendency to go over events leading to the loss and to find someone to blame, even if it means accepting the blame oneself, is a less disturbing alternative than accepting that life is uncertain."[7]

The "if-onlys" can be excruciatingly painful, however, and though they're a normal reaction, it's important to get past them to move forward with the work of grieving.

Finally, many people add to their pain during a period of trouble or loss by judging rather than accepting their many, varied emotions. A misinterpretation of the iconic work of Dr. Kübler-Ross, author of *On Death and Dying*, has contributed to this painful process of devaluing some emotions while prizing others, most specifically "acceptance." The belief that there are set stages to our feelings and that they progress in an orderly way was not the way Kübler-Ross intended her work to be interpreted. As she explained in follow-up works like *Questions and Answers on Death and Dying*,[8] people experiencing traumatic times may notice anger, denial, bargaining, depression, and acceptance recurring in waves that change from day to day, hour to hour, and minute to minute. Expecting an orderly progression or labeling one emotion as more positive than another can only add to our pain, or, if we aren't directly involved in the crisis, will alienate us from others who are experiencing the events. True acceptance of some losses may never be possible, but we may be able to resume our lives, finding meaning and even some joy.

Subsequent to that subdued note, let's move on to our fourth strategy of stress management, step **D**, **D**eciding What to Do.

The first part of deciding what to do involves using some of the information we've looked at in this chapter to diagnose the reason for the stress that you feel. Begin by tuning in to your patterns of thought. Do you sense you're in the throes of a pain-producer? Your pain may range from mild to excruciating, to which anyone who has suffered the demons of self-berating, negative, anxiety-ridden, and otherwise toxic inner tapes can attest.

It's time to take charge of the moment and change the tape, or recording, or channel. Does this concept seem strange? And if so, why should it? If, for example, you were watching a TV show that offended, bored, or annoyed you in any way, no doubt you'd click off almost immediately.

Yet you may not switch off your pain-producing thoughts. Why is this? A lack of awareness, which we've already addressed, is one reason. Habit, the secure sameness of living with these toxic thoughts, is another. After we've developed a habit, no matter how harmful or unpleasant that habit may be, there's a sense of safety in continuing it. It becomes less scary than trying something different and unknown.

Allow me to share an analogy from the world of nature. I am an animal lover and live in South Florida, so it's not unusual to find a small lizard that has slipped in the door to my home. For the purpose of rescuing the reptile and returning it to the outdoors, where it can survive, I keep available a circular strainer with a handle and a large piece of cardboard. First, I capture the lizard under the strainer, which is always tricky because the lizard is terrified and tries to flee. Then I slip the cardboard under the now trapped lizard, go outside, place the cardboard on the ground, remove the upper portion of the "cage," and allow the animal to go free. There is only one problem. The lizard, at first frightened, is now accustomed to the safety of its new environment. When I remove the colander to set it free, the lizard refuses to leave the cardboard floor, remaining frozen although now outdoors and technically free to go. It's now necessary to shake the cardboard vigorously to loosen the lizard, who now feels safe in its former "trap" and is fearful of the unknown. Likewise, our habits of thought and behavior start to feel safe to us. No matter how painful and unproductive they may be, because they're familiar, changing and letting go of those habits seems scary.

Let's look again at figure 3.2. After making a list of some of your most prevalent pain-producers, ask yourself this question: "If I were to want the most nurturing parent/friend/*self* on speed dial to debate this thought, who would I call?" And since we aren't going to actually call, what we're looking for is the most compassionate version of *yourself* we can create—composed perhaps by recollections of kindness in others.

Who would you like on an inner speed dial? Who would you like to call when the world, and *yourself*, were hard on you? Some clients conjure up a parent, usually one who is especially supportive. Some recollect a kind teacher. Others evoke a friend who is empathic.

What's more important than the inspiration, however, is our destination—an inner voice that speaks as an ideally nurturing *self*. That, and that alone, is the strongest antidote to the potential strength of the pain-producing thoughts we all experience at times.

What's needed isn't a harsh response, either. Recriminations such as "How could you be having such a blankety-blank thought? What a stupid thing to do?" is useless in our work. Blaming ourselves for blaming ourselves will only add to our unease. The approach we need is a warm, loving, logical one. It may sound like "Hey, I hear you saying such and such. Let's take a look at reality. You're down on yourself for doing such and such. What was going on for you and what did you see as your actual choices at the time?"

One of the best antidotes for the if-onlys we spoke of earlier is this: "I did the best I could." Yet clients often say to me, "It wasn't the best! If only I'd done such and such my life would be so much better now." To this I offer the amended, even more helpful version of the above rejoinder: "I did the best I could, *given who I was then and what I knew at the time.*"

Suddenly the picture becomes clearer. It's easy to look back and fantasize other, seemingly more perfect choices. But, unfortunately, none of us could have seen the future—the proverbial crystal ball—at the point of decision making. And our hindsight may not be perfect either. For all we know if we'd made the alternate choice, gone, for example, to a different physician, or bought that inexpensive cosmopolitan real estate, perhaps on the way to the doctor's or realtor's we'd have been hit by an intoxicated driver going through a red light!

When we construct our if-onlys, we rarely allow any possibilities that mar our perfect and perfectly pain-producing(!) scenario for the road not taken.

Let's continue with our inner conversation as we discover and discuss those thoughts that feel toxic. Remember to challenge those pain-producers in the same way as would a kind friend. Use logic, compassion, and humor. Be the buddy you'd call or text if you need to switch channels, someone who'd logically, lovingly, and firmly help you embrace reality rather than your pain-tinged habitual style of thought. Picture someone who's on to you but with a smile and a wink!

Let's now take a look at another pain-producer we discussed earlier: incrimination. Suppose we're involved in incriminating, name-calling behavior toward someone in our life, say a spouse. A doubly self-defeating, painful aspect of this behavior is that when we see a friend or a spouse in a totally negative light, who else are we, by inference, berating? Ourselves, of course! That's because we chose to bring and keep this person in our lives. This is the "gift" of blame that keeps on giving—to ourselves, as well as others.

Emma was finally able to catch herself in this cycle after doing some hard work in therapy. A neatness fanatic (who'd grown up in a house full of clutter), Emma was married to John, who loved to be surrounded by papers and knickknacks. He'd been raised in a home in which everything was immaculate and where everyone had to be careful where they breathed. Both Emma and John were expressing their own sense of autonomy by living in conditions visibly different from those of their childhood, but were taking it to an extreme that didn't represent true freedom.

A constant source of contention was their living room coffee table, which always, to Emma, seemed piled high with papers. One day while sitting down on the couch, she took a quick glance at the coffee table and descended into an impotent rage, thinking, "What a jerk. What an SOB! After all our arguments it's still a mess!" Only later did she realize that John had actually removed a lot of the materials and had made considerable progress in decluttering. Because the task wasn't finished, and she was used to feeling fury when she looked at the table, she hadn't allowed herself to see the reality of the situation. Later, she was able to thank John for the improvement and encourage him to continue.

Another pain-producing example involves Maya, who had to go to her stepsister's wedding and swore she "wouldn't be able to stand it" because her stepsister's life was "perfect" and she "always got whatever she wanted." First, together we looked at Maya's life and all that she had accomplished. She finished school and had been working, becoming knowledgeable, sophisticated, and competent in many ways. We explored the way her stepsister's upbringing had hampered her in learning how to face life and the eventual adversities we all face. Maya was eventually able to realize that if she wanted someone for a friend who was caring, open-minded, and intelligent, she, herself, was the best fit because of all she had experienced and the responsibilities she'd handled.

As for the wedding itself, I suggested that she immerse herself in conversations with guests who seemed friendly and really find out, to whatever extent tactful, who they were and what made them tick. There would be far more people there than just her stepsister, so why not find enjoyment with whomever she could, and bring them pleasure as well?

Looking again at figure 3.2, notice how your feelings and mood might have been different if you'd challenged your pain-producing thoughts in a competent, compassionate way. How would the scenario have been different than what we saw in figure 3.1, the pre-CBT picture? Would your feelings and mood have been different, perhaps more calm, more hopeful, and more in control? Would your behaviors have been different? Perhaps a binge would have been avoided. Or might you have reached out to others rather than withdrawn? Perhaps an argument begun by a defensive outburst might have been averted.

So start to uncover your pain-producers, and catch yourself with a smile and a wink—"There I go again. The *old* me! But is that thought really true?" It can be a very helpful technique. Taking charge of our thoughts and becoming that ideal friend/parent/self we'd like in our lives makes a tremendous difference. It takes practice, but it's possible, and well worth it.

A final area that we'll look at in terms of deciding how to relieve our stress is communication. It's easy to see how certain habits of thought that cause pain to ourselves can easily cause pain to others.

One client, a woman named Marge, was experiencing difficulties at work, where she had a high-level professional job. She would frequently come home and overeat after a tough day at her office, where she felt her male colleagues often undercut her. When we explored Marge's behavior and reactions, it soon became apparent that because of her greater academic credentials and experience she was intimidating to her coworkers. When she felt that she was offering helpful criticism, "Your facts are a bit off," she was seen as "castrating" and "not a team player." She had to soften her approach and be more supportive of others in order to get better treatment herself.

Marge, a perfectionist, had grown up in a highly critical family. She had worked hard and longed to be acknowledged by her relatives and professional peers. In Marge's case the thought that she "should" be "heard and respected" distracted her from realizing that others needed to feel appreciated, too. When she softened her tone, offering more respect to others, her work relationships improved accordingly.

If we look back upon potentially stressful situations and see that we overreacted, underreacted, or reacted in a way that was based on a misinterpretation of events, we may need to rectify the situation. Rarely is a sincere apology refused.

Rebekah had been hoping to go out with a fellow in her Spanish class for nearly a year. Whenever she saw him she found it hard to concentrate on her conjugations, and she couldn't help but choose her favorite clothing to wear on the days she'd see him at school. Finally, he texted her for a date, which was, unfortunately, on the same night she'd promised her close friend, Sara, that she'd go out with her and several other friends for Sara's twenty-first birthday. Lacking the courage to ask him to reschedule, Rebekah accepted, but Sara was furious.

Rebekah came to my office very upset because the guy had turned out to be obnoxious and she felt that "if only" she hadn't canceled on Sara, the friendship would be untarnished. Together we looked at Rebekah's background; she was raised in a traditional Jewish family that had always pressured her to "marry well," finding it hard to respect her desire for a career in the arts and to make it on her own. Her parents had been too poor growing up to be able to feel comfortable letting her explore her creativity to see where her talents might lead.

She decided to call Sara and say, "You know how much our friendship means to me and I feel miserable that I may have messed it up. I should have asked that guy to reschedule but I didn't have the nerve. I'm working on respecting myself more in order to be the best possible friend I can be. Spending that special evening with you was something I owed you, and no other person in my life deserved it more than you. Is there anything I can do to make it up to you?" Sara accepted the apology and the friendship resumed, though at first in a somewhat tentative way. It took a while for Rebekah to earn Sara's trust again.

Owning up to mistakes in this way can build character. Not only do I preach this, I do it as well. If I feel a client may have misunderstood me in a way that would be detrimental to their growth, or if I fear I may have inadvertently offended someone, I will try to call as soon as possible to clarify and apologize. If they respond, "No, not at all," I may have been mistaken—although I let the apology stand anyhow. "Not really" indicates that I may have been on the mark in my misgivings—an innocent comment may have been misunderstood—and makes me especially glad that I did make the call.

Very often clients complain that they don't feel they're assertive. Sometimes they're not sure, having lacked sufficient role models, what assertiveness might be. In these cases, I often give this example.

Pretend you're standing in line, at a movie theater perhaps, and someone behind you steps on your foot. The passive response would be to say nothing, while a silent tear falls down your cheek. Nothing is ventured and nothing is gained, except, unfortunately, some anger at yourself that you may experience later. Now let's look at the same situation again. Someone steps on your foot and you shout, "You blankety-blank!" and punch the offender in the nose. That's an aggressive response. We can easily see the downside to that. But what if the same situation arises, and instead you say, "I'm sure you didn't mean to, but you stepped on my foot . . . and it hurt. Please don't do that again." This is an assertive response. You get your point across and usually get results in the form of an apology. It also feels satisfying.

In the past, many of us in the fields of therapy and communication tended to refer to the sandwich technique—a sweet piece of bread (compliment), meat in the middle (the main point you want to get across), and then the final sweet piece of bread (another compliment); but what seems to be most effective to me is an open sandwich. This contains a compliment, the meat of the message, and then a *plan*. If possible, invite the other person to take part—for example, "How can we make our family get-togethers go more smoothly?"

So many people confuse sharing their feelings with "confrontation" or "total honesty" that they're hesitant to make their feelings known at all. This can backfire, causing not only a lot of repressed resentment, but on occasion an explosion of pent-up rage.

Hopefully, this discussion has been productive, and the insights have helped soothe your stress. But if you're still in psychological pain, feeling not only stressed but anxious and depressed, please seek professional help. I myself have done so, completing a personal analysis while I started my career and found it immensely enlightening.

If you're facing an illness or an impending loss, there are many wonderful organizations where you can get individual or group therapy, or which offer support by phone. There are also many wonderful works on coping with loss, including Hope Edelman's *Motherless Daughters*, which has spawned support groups all over the country. Check out the literature on any issue that is causing you concern.

Using the internet to search for organizations that are helpful to people coping with your issue can help you find literature, professionals, and support groups that bring you comfort, insights, and the strength to move forward.

There are many excellent licensed therapists practicing CBT (cognitive behavioral therapy) and DBT (dialectical behavioral therapy)—which is the current name for a softened, slightly more compassionate form of CBT that I practice. Research has shown these techniques are therapeutic in treating stress, anxiety, depression, and more.

The beauty of learning to soothe ourselves—on our own, or with the help of others—is that it enables us to seize the power that food once held for us. By truly understanding our stress, and the ways in which we're vulnerable to causing ourselves additional, unnecessary pain, we become not only stronger, but far freer.

Congratulations! We've now completed the first letter of our one-minute monitor—the letter **S** for Learning from **S**tress. Check in with yourself every day to see how you're doing.

I hope this chapter has been helpful. Now, let's move on.

4

POINT #2: EXERCISE—LEARN TO LOVE IT

We know that movement is a fundamental factor for good health—both mental and physical—as well as longevity. Not only can it lower our blood pressure, but it also lessens our risk of having heart attacks and strokes. Type 2 diabetes, which approximately 30 million Americans are now battling,[1] can be prevented as well as treated by exercise. A study of over 1.4 million people in 2016 indicated a lower risk for thirteen types of cancer—breast, ovarian, and colon, among others—for those who keep active.[2]

A great deal of research also indicates that people who are active experience less depression and anxiety. But those who exercise will often tell you as much. It feels good. After a while, endorphins, our body's "Prozac," kick in, allowing us to have a better attitude about ourselves and our world—to think and plan in a positive way. But in order to get "hooked" on this healthy addiction, it has to happen. And sadly, there's much resistance among the uninitiated.

If you aren't exercising often, you may relate to a recent client's reaction when I introduced the subject. "Oh, no," she said. "I was afraid you were going to bring *that* up! Every therapist I've been to tells me I should but I've tried it and I hate it and I just can't do it. So don't even think about asking me to try it again."

Does this sound and feel familiar? If so, it's probably because exercise has started to feel like a four-letter word to you. No, it's not a sexy word, nor even obscene. On the contrary, it's a word that refers to activities you see as boring and mundane. Exercise not only means "work" to many of us, but work in its most negative nuances. The image evoked is of drudgery and pain (rather than work that might be pleasantly challenging, creative, and self-actualizing), quite different from the way I feel right now as I "work" at writing this, enthused and involved, sitting in a Starbucks, taking in the scene, and listening to New Age music that adds to the ambience. (Not that writing's always easy! More about that later.)

By now you know that exercise isn't only good for you, it's great for you. It can be the key to maximizing and maintaining your mental and physical well-being. That's why it's a crucial component in overcoming emotional overeating. But don't worry; I'll offer no lectures. This approach is about picking up healthy habits and enjoying them—putting the "fun factor" into everything we do.

So how do we adopt this healthy habit?

Let's look back at chapter 2 and the sequence of "cue to routine to reward," and find a way to painlessly apply this principle. Ask yourself how you can transform a cue—one that sent you to your computer, back into bed, or relaxing in front of the TV—into a cue that will get you into your workout wear, out the door, and into an enjoyable activity.

We'll start by turning one four-letter word into another. Think of the word that embodies the polar opposite of work. It's something we rarely put off, never complain about, and often feel our lives are lacking? The word is *play*.

Think back to your earliest remembrances of playing. Savor those memories for a moment. Reexperience the sense of joy and freedom you felt then and now as you relive it. Perhaps your memories, like mine, are of friends knocking on the door and asking you to come outside and play. For me it was kickball in the street. Perhaps for you it was softball, handball, hide-and-seek, or playing on the neighborhood swings. Remember how you felt when the call came or you heard the knock on the door? You were probably excited, dressed in comfortable clothing, and ready to go. What other associations come to mind? You may have been enthused about hanging with your friends, discovering new games, or tweaking existing activities. Perhaps you were looking forward to laughing together, rehashing the day's events at school. Whatever the activities were, you probably did them wholeheartedly—losing yourself in the moment as time flew by. Most likely you were having so much fun you wanted to stay out forever, dreading the call home for dinner.

And now we're at the pragmatic part of our process. Let's brainstorm together to find aspects of this scenario that can be combined with your *current* experience of exercise. Let's change our routine to produce a reward. Use your remembrance to make exercise more enjoyable—less like "working out," more like play, and even fun!

First of all, as a child you were probably playing with people whose company you enjoyed. Is there currently any aerobic activity—tennis, squash, racquetball, handball, hiking, running—that you can enjoy with a group of friends? Perhaps you can sign up for some lessons or clinics or find events where you'll meet other enthusiasts of that activity. Check for local Meetup groups. Google any activities that sound of interest. When it comes to possible sports, the list is endless. What's important is that you give it a try!

If you do get involved in a group activity, be sure to explore what other activities people enjoy. Those game enough to be out and about for sports may also be in the know about other activities and events. Their alternate activity could become your favorite. Even if racing model powerboats isn't aerobic, it's better for your objectives than facing unstructured time in front of the television.

Varying workouts to include both group and individual activities will make it easier to achieve your objective. Why? Because group pressure to show up for a sporting event will help ensure your participation until you're sufficiently involved to want to be there on your own. Again, remember that involvement often precedes interest.

Joining a gym and signing up for classes is a great idea. Many are quite inexpensive and offer different types of movement that you can try until you find the ones you like the most. Many cities offer low-cost classes at community centers or local schools. By going to a group activity, you'll not only meet new people but find that others in your class look forward to your attendance. This creates an expectation that will encourage you to show up.

Let's examine another component of the play mentality we were exploring earlier. Go back to those childhood moments and hear the knock on the door. You were wearing comfortable clothing and couldn't wait to run outside. Unless you grappled with a poor self-image in your childhood, and unfortunately for some of you that may be so, you probably didn't give much thought as to what you were wearing. Your sole concern may well have been comfort.

Unfortunately, for many adults, especially those who are working on emotional eating, the concept of running out to exercise in comfortable clothing, feeling good about their bodies and themselves is foreign. Many new clients tell me they're embarrassed to work out in public or to go to a health club because they're embarrassed about their appearance in activewear. How can we change this mind-set? For me, a positive role model, who incidentally is famous, was helpful, though it's doubtful that she knew it, unless she reads these words.

Years ago, when I was single and living in Manhattan, I was a member of a trendy health club on the Upper East Side. Not only did many of the members look like fashion models and movie stars, they actually were! The handsome man with the flowing blonde hair, huge muscles, and friendly smile who was frequently lifting weights was known as Fabio. Likewise, one day in the ladies' locker room a towel-draped brunette beauty was graciously chatting with all who approached her. Her heavily browed beautiful brown eyes resembled Brooke Shields's for a reason. It was her!

This brings me to the memory of one of the days when I didn't feel at all like going to the club. Instead of thinking about reasons to go and how good I'd feel once I got there, I was focusing only on the fact that I felt overweight (not a size 2!), old (past twenty-one), and unattractive. Though, looking back on that day, I realize that I was a fit young woman, albeit not model-slim nor with a picture-perfect appearance. But comparing myself to all the flashy-looking people at the gym was preventing me from getting to my workout so that I could be the best— inside and out—that I could be.

Realizing this, I dragged myself to the gym, only to see a crowd in the lobby, surrounding a tiny woman wearing a warmup suit and a tremendous, infectious smile. Can you guess who it was? Dr. Ruth! All evening I observed her spread joy wherever she went, attracting more attention and affection than any of the other stars I'd seen in that setting. It wasn't just her fetching, pixie-like demeanor, but also her inner beauty that attracted everyone to her. As I grabbed a salad in the restaurant upstairs, I heard her giggling at a nearby table and informing those around her, "A handsome young man just invited me to a singles' party!"

If you, too, obsess before heading out to a gym or even walking around your block, you can start to make that easier by buying the most comfortable and attractive workout wear you can afford. Make it a treat to sport those outfits as an added incentive to get you on your way. Do you get caught up in the compulsive thought that you should look perfect before you head to the gym or even the street? If so, remind yourself that if you stick with your fitness commitment you'll slowly but surely feel better about how you look. Eventually you may see visible proof of improved fitness, which you'll feel proud to display in your gym attire.

One client, Judy, had the self-defeating habit of examining a roll of fat around her middle as she dressed. Losing motivation, she'd then say to herself, "I'm fat. It's hopeless. Why go to the gym? People are going to judge me for how I look and I won't be able to stand it." We looked together at her behavior as well as her thought patterns of name-calling, negativity, and hopelessness. Together we developed a new plan of action and thought that served rather than sabotaged her efforts.

Although not letting go of her morning "exam," Judy did so less often and allowed herself to notice and enjoy any small improvement she might find. At first she felt an increase in firmness in various parts of her body. She allowed herself to see this and feel proud. She replaced her former thoughts with more positive, encouraging comments, such as, "My body may not be exactly as I'd like it to be, but I'm getting there. I'm working hard and I am starting to see results." Then she noticed the roll of fat for which she had formerly only barraged herself with blame. She realized that it was now a fraction of an inch smaller. For that improvement, she congratulated herself and resolved to stay on track. Reducing her evening eating and keeping on an exercise schedule had been very difficult for her, so seeing this slight improvement was important in maintaining her motivation.

Returning to the play-oriented approach we discussed earlier, what else can we do to keep exercise fun? Since one of the most convenient and healthy exercises for most people is walking, it's definitely worth prioritizing. Walking outside in the country, in a park, by the seaside, even on a tree-lined suburban street can be centering, relaxing, and energizing. A quiet walk can be a perfect opportunity to be mindful, focus on nature, and break free from our ongoing stress.

However, many of us find walking tedious if done in the same place every day. Once while on vacation and visiting a friend in the Northeast, I drove myself fifteen minutes away from her home to another suburban community, just because it was lined by tall, mature trees and looked like a lovely place to walk. Once there I truly savored the beauty surrounding me as I enjoyed the serenity of the canopy created by the towering oaks.

On the just-mentioned trip, another step I took was to join a local gym. You might be surprised to find that there are often temporary, very reasonable two-week, three-week, or one-month memberships if you're out of town and seeking to maintain your fitness. You could easily spend more money in fifteen minutes on an impulse buy at the mall!

Try taking your walking to new terrain. And though walking mindfully, seeing, hearing, and smelling the great outdoors is potentially the most calming and mood-elevating way to go, I'm not a purist. When it comes to moving, do whatever works for you. This may vary from day to day.

How else can we make it more interesting? Do you love music? Do you love to read? Research apps for music you can listen to on your phone. Ride a bike while reading on an e-reader (a stationary bike, that is!). Your public library offers a multitude of music and books available on CDs, as well. If that kind of perk is what it takes to get you on the go, then go for it. But here's another tip. Be firm about not allowing yourself to listen to the music or book anyplace else but during your workout. Otherwise you'll hear that great music, find out "whodunit" in the mystery, or learn the fascinating facts of that famous person's life while driving your car. That won't do much to enhance your health.

What about reading on the treadmill? Some people seem to enjoy it and find that it works out well, but notice the posture of many people who seem to be straining to read a book or a magazine while they walk. Often they're badly hunched over, ignoring the importance of walking with a straight spine, head up, and shoulders back. This puts them at risk for back pain and other health problems. If you want to glance at a book or magazine, you might do best to choose something that's mostly pictorial or try large-print editions or enlarge an article. That way even the slightest bounce while walking won't make it hard to read. Some people enjoy watching television on the treadmill. A physician I know walks daily with his psychologist wife while watching movies they've borrowed from their local library. They delight in the time together while they catch up on classic films.

Ask yourself what else you can do to make your workout less like work and more like fun. Be as creative as you can in varying activities or the place in which you do them. Sometimes I'll walk on a treadmill or use the elliptical at my gym. Other times, I'll walk near my home or change clothing in my office and enjoy the scenic aspects of the area near my work.

Here's another important tip when it comes to being more creative about when and where you exercise. Keep a total workout outfit (i.e., sneakers, shirt, and shorts, plus a change of underclothes) in your car so that you can stop at your gym or sneak in a workout whenever and wherever possible. Granted, this might be more doable if you live in a suburban location and have a slightly more flexible lifestyle. But many of us find that if we stop at home first before going to the gym—even for "just a moment"—we never get out again! Let the momentum of already being out and about carry over to get you wherever you need to go to move. Another option is to take workout clothes with you to work so that you can go directly from work to your gym or a local park for your workout. A locker at your gym would serve a similar purpose. Do anything you can to avoid coming home, where you'll too easily sink into the quicksand of your couch and TV!

Think about the scenario we discussed before. Friends asked you out to play, you rushed out eagerly, becoming so engaged that you lost track of time and maybe even begged to stay out longer—even if it meant eating dinner cold. What were some of the elements that contributed to the ease and pleasure of that activity? I can think of at least four main components that made it playful (perhaps you can think of more). It was easy, creative, convenient, and fun. Contrary to this, many adults set up exercise programs for themselves that are difficult, repetitive, inconvenient, and boring.

Recently I met with a charming retired sales executive who told me that he used to love his work. A "super salesman" with a den whose walls were covered with sales awards, he spoke at length about how he used to customize his approach to suit the unique interests and aspirations of each client. Yet he never thought of using this creativity to make his own exercise program more interesting. He was doing the same thing in the same way five days a week until it became total drudgery.

"Since I retired and started exercising Monday through Friday," he said, "I found out for the first time in my life what TGIF really means!"

If this sounds familiar to you, or inevitable, know that it can be changed. Find a way to vary your exercise activities, as well as when and where you exercise, so that you suit your needs and likes. Choose to intersperse sports, weights, and aerobics so that every day is slightly different. Since a combination of weight training and cardio provide the most benefits for longevity, try a number of different activities combining both.

Also, choose to incorporate intervals into your workout routine. Do whatever activity you're engaged in as vigorously as you can for anywhere from ten seconds to a minute or two. Then hold back and return to your usual level of intensity. Recent studies show that utilizing intervals helps build better strength and endurance, improving your fitness more quickly.

One professional woman I know who is married and the mother of two young children has recently created an innovative and enjoyable program for herself. Early in the morning she does ballet, sometimes utilizing a video. In the evening she does her abdominal crunches. She plays tennis on the weekends and has recently started weekly dance lessons with her spouse. Because she's integrated activities she loves into her program, it doesn't feel like work. The result is that this woman is enjoying herself more than ever as she visibly improves her appearance and fitness.

If you've never exposed yourself to sports, this could be a good time to start. That lost in the moment feeling that we experienced in childhood play is very similar to the feeling of flow that people experience in a competitive sport when they're playing at their best and lose their sense of themselves and of time. I feel it when I'm playing tennis that's competitive and all I think about is the ball and where I want it to go.

If you haven't begun to experience aerobic workouts of twenty minutes or more, you may not have ever felt the pleasure of an endorphin rush. For me it's a combination of calmness, confidence, and optimism, which, once it's ebbed, I crave. This is the feeling that hooks most of us on moving, but it has to happen to become a habit.

By now you may have two pressing questions, especially if you haven't yet started to work out nor experienced the benefits that encourage continuing. Question 1 is, very possibly, "How much is enough?" Or to put it more bluntly, you may be thinking, "How little is enough?" Question 2 is very likely, "What should I do?"

In response, let me be one of the first to inform you that there is good news, and then . . . there is even more good news. Let's start with the first question, "How much is enough?" It's surprising that for over a century, the guidelines have barely budged (pun unintended!).

In 1915 the U.S. surgeon general stated that exercise was "necessary for all except those actually and acutely physically ill, at all ages, daily, in amounts just short of fatigue."[3] Moving up to 1996, the recommendations from the Centers for Disease Control and Prevention (CDC) and the American College of Sports Medicine encouraged thirty minutes of moderately intense physical activity on most, and preferably all, days of the week.[4]

And the CDC guidelines haven't altered over the last twenty years, since they recently advised most Americans to do 150 minutes of moderate aerobic activity each week, plus two muscle-strengthening sessions.[5] Of course, you can exercise longer and at a greater level of intensity, if no physical condition precludes that in your case. But the level and length of workout you require for good health may not be as much as you thought.

What exactly is "moderate aerobic activity" you may be wondering. For most of us it could be walking briskly, swimming, or mowing the lawn. Another option according to the Department of Health and Human Services is seventy-five minutes of vigorous exercise weekly, such as running or aerobic dancing—or a combination of the two throughout the week.

How do you know if you've reached the level of moderate exercise? According to the CDC:

> For moderate-intensity physical activity, a person's target heart rate should be 50 to 70% of his or her maximum heart rate. This maximum rate is based on the person's age. An estimate of a person's maximum age-related heart rate can be obtained by subtracting the person's age from 220. For example, for a 50-year-old person, the estimated maximum age-related heart rate would be calculated as 220 − 50 years = 170 beats per minute (bpm). The 50% and 70% levels would be
>
> - 50% level: 170 × 0.50 = 85 bpm, and

- 70% level: $170 \times 0.70 = 119$ bpm.

Thus, moderate-intensity physical activity for a 50-year-old person will require that the heart rate remains between 85 and 119 bpm during physical activity.

For vigorous-intensity physical activity, a person's target heart rate should be 70 to 85% of his or her maximum heart rate.[6]

Initially you may wish to take your pulse when you exercise, but eventually you'll be able to feel when you're at a moderate or intensive level.

Most exercise physiologists would define moderate exercise as feeling like slightly over a 5 on a scale of 1 to 10, with 10 representing the highest intensity level possible. You can speak, but you'd rather not do so for long. If you cannot speak beware: your level of intensity may be higher than you'd prefer. Chatting in a leisurely way as you walk, however, may well be indicative of a level of activity that won't be sufficiently high to improve your fitness. As President Truman said, "Walk as if you have somewhere to go."

What about jogging? Several years ago my husband and I vacationed at a beach resort thinking at that time that the optimum exercise for me would be to jog two or three times a week, if possible. I mentioned to some of the other guests at breakfast that I was going to go jogging a little later that day. One of the other vacationers, a tall, slim exercise trainer, appearing to be about thirty years old, looked at me in disbelief and said, "You're still jogging? Why don't you come walking with us on the beach? I can't tell you how many jogging injuries I hear about when I go to exercise physiology conferences, and it's frequently people who are in their twenties!" That was one of the first times I rethought my jogging routine, which I truly hated, two or three times a week. If you enjoy running and you have done it without injury, that's your choice, but the chance of injury may be high unless you do it under medical advisement and follow necessary precautions according to your age and level of fitness.

Soon after I switched to walking I started to notice the expressions of the joggers with whom I shared paths. Very rarely did I see a smile. That was one of the reasons I never ran on a regular basis. For me it wasn't fun. I was counting the seconds until I could stop. There was none of the "Hey, Mom, can I stay out and play?" type of feeling that I find in the activities I now fit into my schedule.

Walking also boasts the lowest dropout rate of any form of exercise—no doubt because it's inexpensive, easy, and available for most of us.

Here are some points to remember as you begin a walking routine:

1. Hydrate well. Eight ounces of water every fifteen minutes is ideal if it's hot, but having water handy and sipping often is suggested.
2. Walking faster can help to elevate your HDL (good cholesterol), so consider elevating your heart rate to 65 percent of its maximum (220 minus your age), 55 percent for beginners, for twenty minutes three times a week.
3. Maintain good posture. Think in terms of standing straight, rather than slumping, for the maximum benefits for your spine.
4. Bend your elbows and swing your arms, maintaining them at about chest level.
5. If you jog for intervals, keep your eyes on an object in the distance and try to keep it steady, to maintain a smooth forward motion that will be less jarring on your joints.

What about exercise trackers? Many conversations now seem to start with the question, "Have you done your ten thousand steps yet today?" When they first came out, exercise trackers seemed to be the answer to our nation's issues with inactivity and the resulting high rates of obesity. However, a recent study in *The Lancet: Diabetes and Endocrinology*, which studied eight hundred people living in Singapore, aged twenty-one to sixty-five, did not find any significant health benefits from the devices.[7] In the Singapore study, the participants were separated into four groups: a control group without a tracker; a group that was given a Fitbit device; and two final groups, one of which was given cash for upped activity, while the other had donations given to charity in their name. Weekly moderate to vigorous physical activity was tracked as well as cardio fitness, both at the study's start, and six and twelve months afterward. The score of steps daily was 11,010 for those receiving cash, 9,280 for those donating to charity, and 8,550 for those wearing a Fitbit.

Those getting cash reverted to their former levels of exercise in one year. Those wearing the Fitbit did increase their exercise time by sixteen minutes, and didn't show the same decline as those who received neither a device nor a cash incentive, but still, the conclusions of the researchers were that the results were probably not enough to generate noticeable improvements in any health outcomes.[8]

Most recent studies, including one published in the *Journal of the American Medical Association* (JAMA), indicate that the effectiveness of the fitness tracker depends on the innate motivation of the individual. They can't make you exercise unless you really want to.[9]

The only magic button to turn us on to exercise is our brain. Again, you need to find something you like to do, and do it often enough, and intensely enough, that eventually, liking may even turn to love. First, find one or more weight-bearing aerobic activities you can do most days of the week for at least one half hour per day. You'll then add weight training at least two days a week. Why do both? Aerobic exercise requires a lot of oxygen and stimulates production of the aerobic enzymes, which helps burn fat. Weight training helps to increase your muscle mass. Since muscle cells burn calories more effectively than fat cells, this will also increase your metabolism.

"But I hate to exercise!" you may be saying. "I'm tired of hearing all these skinny people talking about how much they love to work out. It doesn't do a thing for me." We've talked about the difference between work and play. The first means doing something you don't want to do. The second involves having fun and doing something you not only like, but *love*. If the words *exercise* or *working out* have negative connotations for you, ask yourself a new question: "I know I need to move more. How can I do that by doing what I already love to do?" Then ask yourself what those activities might be.

Do you love to read? As we noted before, you can listen to a book on your phone or on tape while you walk outside or on the treadmill.

Do you love to dance? Take a class in aerobic dance, Jazzercise, Zumba, or ballroom dancing.

Do you love animals? Walk with your dog, or, if you don't own one, and space and time permit, adopt one—most breeds and many uniquely adorable mixes are available in local shelters; you can also check out petfinder.org for an initial view online. You may notice that many of the humans seen out walking are attached to the leash of a pup proudly leading them on a stroll.

Research at Purdue University in 2015 found that dog owners given material about the benefits of exercise not just for themselves but for their pets subsequently walked farther than a canine-owning control group—extra minutes of walking that added up to real health benefits.[10] These results have been replicated elsewhere in similar studies.

In his highly informative *How Not to Be My Patient*, Edward T. Creagan, a cancer specialist at the Mayo Clinic, lauds the curative powers of pets. In his subchapter "There's Something about a Wagging Tail,"[11] he speaks about the endorphins released when we stroke our pets, their ability to lower our blood pressure, how they encourage us to move, and why they can help ward off depression. This gives deeper meaning to the "Who saved who?" stickers, written on a paw print, that are currently popular on the backs of vehicles. (Perhaps your "fitness tracker" needs a wagging tail and a wet nose!)

Whether or not a canine's in your future, you may have other preferences that could help make movement fun. Do you love being with others? Play a social sport like tennis, which offers the added benefit of knowing that others are waiting for you, requiring your presence to have a game, so it's unlikely you'll back out. You could also enlist a friend or friends to walk with you, but be sure that your pace is brisk enough so that it isn't easy to chat while you're walking. Otherwise, you won't get the full aerobic benefit.

Do you like to watch TV? You could place your exercise equipment in front of the television, or work out with free weights to music videos. Most gyms and exercise facilities now have TV screens embedded in the equipment so it's easy to mix your exercise with tube time.

Are you into fashion? Treat yourself to the trendiest workout wear you can find. Since these clothes no longer go only to the gym—"athleisure" is the current nomenclature—you can rationalize the expenditure as weekend wear, recreational wear, and almost-wherever wear. Tell yourself that as you get fitter you'll be able to buy even more exciting and revealing styles.

Do you love the great outdoors? Take up biking, rowing, hiking, or skiing. Intersperse this with other activities you can engage in even more regularly. When you develop a passion for a sport you'll discover that you want to improve your fitness to achieve peak performance.

There are many different options. The number of aerobic and strength-training techniques seems to be expanding all the time, from the ancient yet never trendier than today tai chi, to the technologically dependent recent rage for spin. Glance through the following list of options and see what intrigues you. Try several, and give each activity more than one chance, since a mediocre instructor may turn you off to an activity that you'd really love if you tried it under other circumstances.

Aquatic Exercises—If you want to place minimum stress on your joints, this could be a good activity for you. It's also helpful for cardio fitness and for use after an injury. Rather than swimming you'll be doing exercises while in the water, in a relatively upright position, usually with music playing to add to the fun.

Barre—This utilizes fluid movements and works to help you develop long, lean muscles. Imagine yourself aspiring to achieve the grace of a ballerina as you move to beautiful music.

Bicycling/Stationary Cycling—This is easy on the joints and can be done indoors or out, but it's important to take safety measures when biking outdoors, especially in large cities where you're mingling with other traffic. Since biking clubs are popular this can also be a very social activity.

Cardio Boxing—A wonderful way to achieve high-intensity exercise while releasing any aggression you're bottling up inside! It's fun, and potentially therapeutic, both for body and mind.

Hiking—This is an excellent cardiovascular and muscular workout utilizing practically all of the muscles in your body. As with all outdoor exercises, you can also benefit from the serenity of nature, which has been shown to aid in lessening depression. But hiking doesn't always have to be done on an exotic trail. If there's a hill near your place of work, on a break you can hike that, too, and enjoy similar benefits.

Jazzercise—This exercise was launched in a YMCA gym in 1972 by a professional dancer and it quickly rose in popularity. The classes usually involve a warmup, aerobic exercise, strength training with weights, and then stretching to cool down. The classes are now so prevalent that there may well be one near you!

Pilates—This exercise focuses on the importance of centering and an awareness that all of our bodily movements begin in our core (our abdominal and trunk muscles), which is strengthened by this training. It was developed about one hundred years ago in New York by Joseph Pilates and was first used by ballet dancers seeking better posture and control of their bodies. It's best to learn it in a class, as the proper form is important to avoid injury. Some studios teach Pilates using equipment, but Mat Pilates is also popular.

Power walking—As you may have noticed, I'm personally partial to walking, and if you'd like to ramp it up a notch, power walking may be right for you. Potentially burning almost the same calories as running, power walking is characterized by an unusual hip movement allowing continuous contact between the feet and the ground. The elbows are also pumped in an arms-up position. Other variations on traditional walking include walking hills, jogging at intervals, or using light hand weights.

Running—Always run or walk in daylight and against traffic. Be aware of the possibility of vehicles and cyclists at intersections. If you're wearing headphones or other devices to listen to music, be sure to have the volume low enough so that you can hear sound around you that might indicate approaching vehicles and other dangers. As there are numerous clubs, and marathon events, the latter often supporting charities, running can be a highly social, even humanitarian activity. Be aware, though, that it can be stressful to your joints.

Rowing—Using a rowing machine provides great exercise for muscles in both the upper and lower parts of your body and improves both aerobic and muscular fitness. Most gyms now offer them. There's little stress to your joints if you row correctly.

Sex!—Surprise! I bet you never expected to find this here. Yes, what can be the most sensual, spiritual, loving, and uplifting experience known to humankind is also calorie burning, stress relieving, and a lot of fun! If you don't have a loving significant other, please consider choosing someone you know and trust, someone you care about and who cares about you. And yes, that can even be yourself! Even if you fault your body for not being picture perfect (whatever that may be), learning the pleasure your body can give you may help you appreciate it more. If you've never experienced the joy of orgasm, a wonderful classic titled *For Yourself*, by Lonnie Barbach, is worth checking out. And remember, let your fantasies run wild. They are your own. There's no need to judge or censor. Allow yourself—and, if possible, your partner—this precious opportunity to soothe and self-soothe.

Skating—Roller-skating (as mundane as this may seem after the former suggestion!) can offer a total aerobic workout, utilizing most, if not all, of your body's muscles, including your heart. It's comparable to running in terms of its benefits to your health, calories burned, loss of body fat, and so on. Ice-skating offers similar benefits depending on how hard you skate. Both build leg muscles and enhance balance.

Skiing—If you don't mind the cold and some height, and for some of us this sport has changed our attitudes toward both, this could be a great activity for you. Skiing can strengthen your knees and your bones, improve your cardiovascular fitness, increase your balancing ability and core strength, as well as increase your flexibility. As with any new activity, instruction is important at the beginning, and safety measures should be observed.

Snowshoeing—This is a form of hiking in which the latticework on the sole of your shoes creates a form of flotation so that you don't sink into the snow. Studies show that it burns more calories than running or cross-country skiing, and it's definitely an excellent cardio workout that develops greater strength, endurance, and balance. Minimal equipment is required.

Spin—Some people consider this to be bicycling on steroids, but you can choose to make your workout less intense if desired. Little equipment is needed. Cycling shoes are advised if you take to the activity, but they aren't immediately essential. Loud and lively music helps create an energizing atmosphere.

Squash—This fast-paced racquet sport is most often found in major cosmopolitan areas, where it packs in quite a punch of highly aerobic, exciting exercise in minimum time with minimal equipment. But joining a club may be a requirement. Otherwise, court time may be charged by the hour. Attending parties where you can meet potential partners is one good way to meet fellow devotees.

Swimming—It's an excellent way to get and keep in shape that can be practiced for a lifetime. You can try various strokes (butterfly, crawl, freestyle, breaststroke, and backstroke) or tread water, which also expends calories. Alone or combined with other exercises, it's great for fitness, although there's been some recent controversy as to whether it's effective for weight loss, given that it doesn't raise body temperature.

Yoga—This highly ritualized activity originated in India and is considered more than exercise by those who think of yoga as a way of life. Not only can it improve your flexibility, your strength, and body tone, you may also find that it enhances your physical and emotional well-being. I find the classes calming. Both the poses and the soothing words of the instructor often help to clear my mind from any concerns I'm coping with that day. Many different forms of yoga are available, some in gyms and health clubs, others at yoga centers. They include

- *Hatha*, a combination of poses, meditation, and breathing that serves to achieve a better balance between body and mind.
- *Vinyasa*, a way to get in some good stretches, tone up, and achieve better balance—all while achieving a greater sense of both vigor and calm.
- *Ashtanga*, a combination of various poses, along with what is referred to as heated breath. Since the movement between poses is continuous, this form can be more demanding.
- *Bikram*, similar to Ashtanga but is practiced in a heated area. Some people love it, but others find the ambience too uncomfortable.

Try experimenting with different types of beginner classes if you're a newbie and see which style of yoga suits you best. Visit various gyms, fitness centers, and studios until you find your yoga home.

Zumba—a high-energy workout incorporating Latin dance moves, hip-hop, or a combination of the two. Instructors usually practice their own unique style. Because of the happy, dance-party ambience, it can easily become the most fun you'll ever have with your clothes on!

For many of the above activities joining a gym or community center can be especially helpful, since professional trainers will be available to assess your abilities and guide you along the way. And just because you work with a professional doesn't mean you need their presence every time you work out. Many athletic individuals simply ask for a program that they can do on their own—including aerobic activity and strength training—and then meet periodically with the trainer to tweak the routine as needed. Be sure to voice your preferences for the types of activities you like to do. Otherwise you'll end up with a repertoire that's easy to avoid.

Speaking of which—one common exercise excuse is "I don't have the time!" This is a common cop-out and often becomes an easy excuse for inactivity. My favorite response to this statement comes from a timeless tome on time management, *Getting Things Done*, by Edwin C.

Bliss. Noting that even Fortune 500 CEOs can find thirty minutes a day to exercise, he admonishes,

> If you are too busy to exercise, you are too busy. In your hierarchy of values, nothing can have higher priority than health, and if you find time for watching television but not for tennis or golf or jogging, you are violating the most basic rule of time management, which is to do the most important things first.[12]

So take a look at all of the less "essential" activities you somehow find time for in your day—watching TV, surfing the net, texting mindlessly, windowshopping, and the like. Yes, these pastimes have their place, but when they replace essential, life-saving activity, it's time to reassess.

Just as you'd schedule, on your phone or on paper, an appointment with a pal, make a date with yourself to improve your fitness and health. Ask yourself when you're most likely to make it happen. For most of us, first thing in the morning, before others get a chance to interrupt our day, rescheduling it to suit their purposes, is the best time to set our priorities.

Another powerful reason to prioritize exercise in the morning is that this will shift your biorhythms into more of a morning through early evening pattern. New research reconfirms that eating a hearty meal earlier in the day, less at lunch, and our smallest meal in the evening, mirroring the old adage many of us have heard since childhood, contributes to more effective weight control. In the largest study of its kind, published in *The Journal of Nutrition*, July 2017, researchers studied fifty thousand adults and found that to keep weight in check the timing and frequency of meals is a significant factor.[13] Eating more than three meals a day, skipping breakfast, and eating heavier meals later in the day were all associated with higher body mass index (BMI).

"Eat breakfast like a king, lunch like a prince, and dinner like a pauper," Dr. Hana Kahleova, a researcher at the Loma Linda University School of Public Health, commented in a press release for the study.

Although this study indicated that the gain in weight was due to increased eating, similar studies show that metabolic changes can result in greater BMI regardless of caloric intake, a somewhat surprising result. But however you interpret the results, you may now agree that those of us who are prone to emotional eating are better off with less unstructured time at home. Eating less in the evening will also help prevent the discomfort of a condition called reflux, for which one of the contributing factors is a pattern of eating and drinking heavily shortly before bedtime.

Nevertheless, if exercising in the morning is impossible, choose another alternative that's convenient for you, perhaps your lunch hour (if fitness facilities and a shower are available) or in the evening immediately after work. It's key at first, before the habit's taken hold, to record it in your schedule, to ensure that nothing that seems more pressing precludes it. Allow yourself to feel good about keeping a date with yourself, and for believing you deserve to be treated well.

"What if I don't feel like it?" This excuse is an interesting and often informative catch-22. Because whenever we feel least like exercising is usually when we need it most.

At one point during the writing of this book I found a mind-boggling error in my method of counting the words I'd written. As a result, I was short by twenty thousand words! That's a lot of writing. Within a week I was able to add another eight thousand words, but only on aspects of this work that were mostly psychological and therefore second nature to me. Aspects that were further afield and required more research were yet to come.

This was very stressful. A number of tyrannical shoulds and terribilizing thoughts kicked in and I didn't feel good at all. As a result, I woke up one morning thinking that the last thing I felt like doing was going to the gym. If I hadn't been the writer of this book (and therefore a motivational "maven"!), I'd probably have simply pulled up the covers, slept some more, or tried to hide out from the world. But my sense was that I would benefit most from doing exactly what I wanted most to avoid—exercise. And do you know what? Soon thereafter, not only these thoughts, but others relevant for clients and myself emerged into my consciousness. These seemed to enter my awareness serendipitously, as I strode the elliptical, glancing back and forth between clouds in the sky outside and a rock video I was watching on the screen.

Remember your priority, whenever possible, to treat yourself well. A healthy mind and body is your right. Reclaim it. The feeling that we don't deserve to treat ourselves well is a deterrent to many would-be exercisers.

Janet, a forty-five-year-old client, had been molested by her step-father. She found that she could "disappear" by being fat as an adult, thereby escaping much male attention. Eating mindlessly, at meals and afterward, soothed her, since it distracted her momentarily from her shame and pain. But the extra weight only left her feeling worse about herself, driving her to crave the numbness of overeating even more. She had to make peace with herself, forgiving herself for her former help-lessness, before she could employ more effective means of coping with stress—including exercise.

Another example of opting out when we need it most is connected to a special type of stress. During the illness of a loved one, "survivor's syndrome"—guilt at being healthy—can kick in. One client I recall, an athletic-looking man of sixty, had a wife with advanced cancer who required and received round-the-clock professional help at home. When I asked how he kept so fit, he answered, "I bike. But am I still allowed to do that?" You can guess how I answered. But we also had to have a longer discussion of what survivor's syndrome is about, that there isn't just one big pie of health, life, and happiness from which we're stealing a piece if we survive. Intellectually we may know it's true, but emotionally we may not accept that, especially if we're living with a loved one who's ill.

Another deterrent can be perfectionism. If you miss a day, don't dwell on it. Learn from what went wrong, so you can tweak your sched-ule the following day, improving your priorities. Aiming for "most days" will help prevent a sense of failure when your workout doesn't work out! Review what happened to better prevent it from happening again.

You now know the meaning of the letter **E** in "Am I doing what's best for my **SELF**?" Yes, it's **E**xercise, and you're asking yourself if you've done it that day. If you're tuning in to the tips above, you're well on your way to answering, "Yes!," and feeling better as you become as active as you can be. Both your mind and body will benefit.

Be aware of what helped get you moving. Make sure to do more of whatever worked. Congratulate yourself on your efforts!

5

POINT #3: LOVE YOUR FOOD—HANDS-ON TECHNIQUES

You're ready now for a key component of *Love Your Food*—hands-on techniques. We'll begin with a restaurant meal, because it eliminates the added elements of making and serving the food and it's also a setting in which many of my clients report they overeat. The goal at this meal, as at all of your meals, is to truly enjoy your food, to "be there" in the moment, and be totally satisfied without overeating.

As you're learning to love your food, choose to eat whatever tempts you (barring allergies or strict medical prohibitions from your physician). The beauty of intuitive, nonrestrictive eating is that it frees us to choose whatever we please. When all foods are allowed, our former "forbidden" foods lose their unique allure. We're then free to find new favorites and eventually enjoy the appeal of new more nutritious fare.

For your first *Love Your Food* eating experience, it's best to lunch or dine alone or with a pleasant, easygoing partner at a restaurant with an attractive and restful ambience. Advanced practitioners of *Love Your Food* can use these techniques anywhere, even in a fast-food restaurant with several restless toddlers in tow.

Whether it's lunchtime or dinnertime, you may be feeling frazzled by the frantic pace of your day. Whether dashing about the workplace, dealing with the demands of child rearing, juggling roles as caregiver, spouse, or whoever else, many of us seem to be rushing around multitasking. Our preoccupation with our constantly changing, unpredictable universe and our current compulsion to stay connected only compound our stress.

Meals, however, are a time to forget as many of these chores and challenges as possible. Turn off your cell phone, laptop, iPad, and so on. Tune out your concerns and think only of tuning in to relaxing and loving your food.

Dare to disconnect? For many of us this concept may seem scary. We're so hooked on Facebook, Twitter, Instagram, or whatever the internet addiction of the moment might be that it's hard to imagine eating a meal without it. Yet studies show that there's a correlation, a distinct association if not a proven cause and effect, between the amount of time spent on social media and levels of depression. So tune out your devices, and tune in to your own delight at satisfying your hunger and savoring your food.

THE RAFT TECHNIQUE

At this point I'm going to introduce an acronym and image, which will help you visualize how mealtime should feel. Remember the four steps involved. The acronym is **RAFT**, for **R**elaxation, **A**wareness, **F**ullness Check, and **T**aking Charge of the Moment. As the word suggests, imagine yourself drifting away from the tensions of your day and allowing yourself to truly enjoy the mental and sensual excursion a meal can be. You're now about to "embark" on step 1.

Relaxation

It's time to relax for your meal. Is there any best way? Perhaps you have favorite techniques of your own. If not, I'll suggest some of mine.

What's most important about this step, however, isn't how well you do it, but that you're doing it at all! Why? Because believing that it's time to slow down, take it easy, and enjoy your food is very foreign from the feelings most of us have today in our frenetic, fad diet–obsessed, food-fearing culture. You're saying yes to yourself and no to unnecessary tensions—a behavior you'll learn here and then extend elsewhere when applicable.

Take a deep breath and tell yourself that it's time to sit back, relax, and enjoy your meal. As you're doing so, actually lean back, allowing the small of your back to rest against the back of your chair. Notice how this feels. Now briefly close your eyes and inhale through your nose with your mouth closed, counting silently to five. Then exhale through your mouth, letting the tension seep from your body as you let your breath unfold. Count to eight as you exhale. As you continue with your meal allow your belly to expand as you inhale and contract as you exhale. You might press your hand upon your stomach to feel it rising and lowering as you breathe. This is called diaphragmatic, yoga, or belly breathing, and is both healthy and relaxing.

Another great tension breaker is the "rag doll"—a favorite of professional public speakers who use it just prior to starting a speech. Let your body lean forward slowly and gently until your upper half is hanging loosely. Then slowly and gently feel first your spine, then your head rise upward, as if elevated by invisible strings attached from high above and hanging down to your head and shoulders. If you feel uncomfortable doing this in a public place, place your purse or a laptop on the floor beside you and do the stretch subtly as you lift your belongings.

Head rolls can also be quite relaxing. Sit back in your chair, which I realize might seem a strange sensation to some of you while at the table, and let your head slowly hang forward as you take a nice long breath. Feel the soothing stretch at the back of your neck. Let your head roll gently to the right, feeling the stretch on the opposite side of your neck and the opposite shoulder; return to the center and then to the left. Keep your shoulders relaxed and your arms hanging loosely by your sides.

Finish whichever exercise you chose by turning away from the table, if necessary, then leaning back, raising your arms straight out in front of you, clasping your fingers lightly together, and feeling the gentle pull on your shoulders and upper back.

Pick your favorite, but most importantly *do it*. It's time to take a break from the day's demands and to relax.

Awareness

You're now ready for step 2. Look at your surroundings and notice whatever engages or appeals to you as your gaze drifts slowly around the room. Allow yourself to settle in and observe the pleasant aspects of the setting, such as fresh, fragrant flowers on the table, a scenic view, even attractive features of the people around you. Perhaps your lunch companion has gorgeous green eyes or is wearing a tie that's a pleasing paisley print. Feast your eyes on your surroundings as you focus on whatever attracts you. Likewise let whatever disturbs or distracts you "drift" by. Be selfishly selective about what you allow to seize and hold your attention.

As you do so, check to see if there's a glass of water available, and if not, request one. As you drink, continue to "feast" on the lovely, soothing sights around you. As the meal progresses, take sips of your water whenever possible, leaning back in your seat, and relaxing as you do. Try to drink at least one glass of water prior to the meal and another glass as you eat.

While you're savoring your surroundings, leaning back, relaxing, and awaiting the menu, there may be an emotional intrusion—an unpleasant thought or concern connected to your harried day or an ongoing issue in your life. Note this as something you may wish to deal with at *another* time and then, most important, allow it to drift away.

Now it's time to take a look at the menu. As you glance at the offerings, ask yourself, "Exactly what would I like to eat?" What do you crave most at this moment? Is it something rich and creamy? Or would you like something crunchy? Would it be warm or cold? Perhaps something light like a salad appeals to you? Or maybe you long for a dish that's heavier and more rapidly filling?

Make your choice and let your imagination soar. Begin to enjoy your selection even before it arrives. Picture whatever you've chosen at its peak pleasure-giving potential. A hamburger? If that's your inclination, imagine it in the manner that would be most appetizing to you—perhaps hot, pink in the middle, oozing flavorful juices and seared on top, as it would be right off of a barbecue grill.

An omelet? How do you picture the additions? What kind of cheese? Mushrooms? Onions? Fries on the side? What exactly would their shape and texture be?

Perhaps it's a fish filet that's caught your fancy. Would it be flakey yet moist, blackened or broiled, flavorful yet not overly fishy?

Veggies? Would they be grilled or sautéed? Do you prefer them al dente or soft in texture? Do you imagine them brilliantly, boldly colorful and fresh?

After you've ordered, sit back, relax, and continue to entertain fantasies of the wonderful meal you're about to enjoy.

Fullness Check

Now you're ready to try another technique you'll be using several times at every meal: a fullness check. Tune in once more to your body, this time to get a sense of exactly how hungry you feel.

Picture a scale of 1 to 9, with 1 representing the hungriest you've ever felt, perhaps after a fast or another occasion when food was unavailable and the result was pain, weakness, and fatigue. A 9, on the other hand, would represent an instance when you overate to the point of feeling painfully full, nauseous, and even wished to vomit. A 5 is the point at which you feel perfectly satisfied: more food might still provide pleasure, but on another level you realize it's not physically necessary that you continue to eat.

As you await the arrival of your order, ask yourself how your level of fullness rates on this scale of 1 to 9. If you're aware of physical distress, such as stomach contractions, you may actually be at a 2. If you just feel enthusiastic about eating and have a slight sense that you are hungry—a vague, slightly empty feeling throughout your body that's hard to trace—you may be at a 3 or a 3.5. Don't fret about perfection in rating your fullness. Realize that tuning in to your level of need for food is a new and very positive step for you.

Perhaps you sense that you aren't at all hungry, but the offerings on the menu look alluring anyhow. You'd do best to postpone your meal for an hour or so, but if you choose to eat now, do the *Love Your Food* eating experience another time so you'll gain more from it.

Continue to sip your water as you wait for your meal. Lean back and allow yourself to bask in a sea of pleasurable sensations, casting off all your troubles and allowing them to drift away. Perhaps you'll choose to recapture any concerns of the day at another time, when you aren't eating and can deal with them in a purposeful, productive way.

As you're leaning back, relaxing, and sipping, the server may place a tray of bread or rolls at your table. If you like bread and have no health issues with eating it, go ahead and have some. It happens to be one of the most filling foods, calorie for calorie, that you can eat and, in spite of its oft-maligned image, isn't calorie intensive. So scan the tray of bread or rolls and ask yourself which item looks most appealing. I love piping hot bread, smelling like it's fresh from the oven, firm and crusty outside yet fluffy inside. If you like your bread with butter, allow yourself a small pat. Immerse yourself in the experience of that hearty slice of bread or roll, savoring its warmth if it's hot, as well as its scent, taste, and texture. Take another sip of water as you lean back. Continue to enjoy the sights, sounds, and scents surrounding you, including the doughy delight of your choice.

By now you should have finished your first glass of water and your meal has arrived. Take a deep breath and peruse your platter. Is it what you expected? Perhaps the presentation is lovely. In that case, enjoy it. Notice the color of the plate, the decorative swirls of cream or sauce, the garnish, or whatever else looks appealing. Take a whiff of any aromas emanating from the dish. What are they? Do they enhance your anticipation of the enjoyment you'll experience?

On the other hand, does your dish disappoint? Is your medium-rare burger well done, the egg undercooked? Is the salad missing some of the additions listed on the menu? Then beckon the server and seek solutions. It's your meal, you're paying for it, and you have every right to enjoy it.

Now that you've enjoyed the sight and scent of your selection, lean back and take your first bite. If you're somewhat hungry and your selection's close to your expectations in terms of taste, texture, and scent, it's likely that you're loving your food right now! Savor each bite slowly as you sip your water. Between each bite set down your silverware and sit back in your seat.

Tune in to what's enjoyable about your experience. What surprises and delights you? I remember, for example, a wonderful soup I had not long ago, a carrot purée that was hot, festively pumpkin colored, and fragrant with freshly minced spices. I realized that it reminded me of Thanksgiving—a holiday whose sights and scents evoke some of the most cherished memories of my childhood. Likewise, let yourself notice what's novel or nostalgic about the sight, scents, and tastes of your selection.

Not long ago I sampled a vanilla-flavored milk at our local supermarket. Loving it, but not knowing why, I took some home and sat in my kitchen savoring it. Suddenly a recollection of childhood came back to me in which I was at a lunch counter finishing a vanilla malted only to be told by the kindly counterman, "There's more, little girl. Here, have what's left." The cool, vanilla milk reminded me of my favorite part of the shake, the leftover portion, and the kindliness with which it was offered. It's reassuring to realize that we can revisit and relish such recollections whenever we choose. Allow yourself to get in touch with pleasing associations. It can enhance your pleasure and serendipitously soothe you, as well.

Have you ever noticed the joy with which some children eat? Why not also allow yourself to toy with your food, as kids often do? Say, for example, that you've ordered french fries. Notice their texture and shape. What's your preference? I like steak fries, large, thickly rectangular, and well done. Perhaps you'd like to cut one fry in half and dip it into a sauce that came with your dining partner's order. Enjoy experimenting with different tastes and combinations. With your friend's permission, explore and have fun.

Another trait many youngsters share is their tendency to eat exactly what they like, sparing the rest. They may order a slice of pizza and chomp away at the first few cheesy mouthfuls, leaving the crust uneaten because they like it less. Likewise, allow yourself to eat only what really pleases you.

Not long ago I ordered an apple crisp a la mode, which my server said was outstanding. It arrived a good fifteen to twenty minutes later, hot and bubbling in a china tureen. Emanating from the dish were the fresh bakery aromas. I could see myself, as a child, standing in line behind my mother, smelling freshly baked butter cookies, one of which I was invariably offered as we waited. In contrast to the apple crisp's piping hot crust, the vanilla ice cream was cold and silky, yet similarly sweet, melting rapidly over the crust and apple combination just below. I adored every bite of the crust and ice cream, but not the apple filling, so I left some of that uneaten, aiming to satisfy my hunger and appetite only with what I really loved.

Returning again to your eating experience, ask yourself whether anything on your friend's plate looks appealing. Ask if they would like to sample your dish. Should that be the case, ask if you might try a taste of theirs.

Now's the time to take your second fullness check. What number have you reached? Are you approaching a 4 or a 4.5? That means that you're going to reach satiety soon. Another clue that you're approaching fullness is that you're *liking* your food rather than *loving* it. The bloom is off the rose. Allow yourself to tune in to these feelings. If you're still enjoying your food but the physical feelings of hunger have passed, you may be approaching a crucial point of your meal, the moment of fullness.

Taking Charge of the Moment

If much of what you've read in the previous paragraph feels true, if the food on your plate now looks appealing but not compellingly attractive and your previous feelings of hunger have been satiated, tune in to this change. It signals that you may be approaching an all-important moment. You've *loved* your food, *liked* your food, and, yes, now it's time to *leave* your food. You're at a 5, perfectly satisfied. You need no more, and—best of all—you know it!

Allow yourself another bite or two. Then acknowledge that you've just become full and that it's time to stop eating. (You may opt, however, to order some coffee or tea to sip as you spend some additional time relaxing and chatting with your companion.)

What does the experience at this point feel like for you? Yes, it's truly momentous and you'll have to be fully aware of it, even embrace it, if you're going to take charge of your eating, your weight, and, to some degree, your life. But watch for some of these emotions you may be experiencing at the end of your meal.

> *Sadness.* This and a sense of loss are feelings many clients have reported and which at this point in a meal I've experienced myself. There's a sense of mourning the past pleasures of the eating experience coupled with worry that the pleasures to follow during that day or evening won't compare to those that have transpired.
>
> *Disappointment.* The much-anticipated meal, which was delicious, is now over.
>
> *Anger.* You paid for the food and have every right to eat it.

Guilt. "That leftover food on my plate could feed starving children."

Allow yourself these feelings. It's important to be aware of your personal pattern of thoughts at this momentous point of your meal.

Now, take a final fullness check. If you're sure you're at no more than a 6, satisfied but not yet experiencing any unpleasant sensations of feeling overly full (pain, tight clothing, or gastric distress), put down your utensils, call over your server, and ask that your plate be taken away.

Congratulations! You've taken charge of the moment, the meal, and yourself. As time goes on you'll master these techniques as you launch a lifelong habit of eating and enjoying a healthy variety of foods in sensibly sparing portions.

Yes, you're experiencing intense emotions after eating a meal in this new and different way. Some may be positive. Others may not. If so, don't despair! Any change can be challenging. Although the *Love Your Food* eating experience was probably pleasurable, you may sense some distress, as well.

Since your reaction to the experience may afford important insights for further self-growth let's look more closely at some of the emotions that are frequently elicited.

As stated before, these may include a sense of disappointment, sadness, and loss. Yes, it may seem a shame that every meal must end, but if these feelings are intensely painful, you may need to work on other aspects of your life. One possibility is that there are other losses you haven't given yourself permission to fully mourn.

In the absence of a loss, ask yourself, "What has made it hard to allow myself other food-free pleasures?" Explore the reasons and start now to schedule more fun in your life. This will help lessen the letdown feeling you have at the end of a meal. If you're still reluctant to curtail your eating, consider, as a "perk," how good you'll feel embarking on your day or evening feeling light and energetic, rather than heavy, stuffed, and sluggish.

Another way to ease the pain of ending a meal is to ponder how fantastic you'll feel the next time you eat. If you forego overeating you'll approach your next meal with an excellent appetite, all the more able to re-create the exhilarating experience of loving your food again! Isn't that exciting to anticipate?

You might also experience some anger, which is valid. You paid for the food and have every right to eat it! But cleaning your plate when you're no longer hungry will cheat you in the long run, impairing your health and overall enjoyment of life. Is that worth the small amount of money you might "save"? (Also, you can take some food home, or give it to the homeless, which I do if I'm staying in a fridge-free hotel room.)

Ask yourself about the sources of this anger. Does it remind you of your childhood when you were faced with parents who were overly strict regarding eating or other issues? Revisit those painful periods and the ways in which you coped regarding this and other issues. Maybe some of those coping mechanisms were productive while others were not. Remind yourself that as an adult *you* can be in charge, not just of what you eat, but also of when you choose to start and stop eating. When you stop as an adult it's not because you were forced to by someone else. It's because you're satisfied, your enjoyment of food has ceased, and you care too much for yourself to continue and overeat.

Many of us suffer from middle-class guilt and angst. We're living well and wish that everyone else could, too. Perhaps our parents had struggled at some point financially and frequently reminded us of our privileged status. If this rings true for you, think of those times. Feel your own pain and show yourself compassion now.

One client, Karen, had been the youngest of four siblings in a wealthy household. She'd been called a "rich bitch" throughout her childhood by her parents, who'd been raised in poverty. It was almost impossible for her to leave any uneaten food on her plate. In working together I had to help Karen relive those painful experiences and regain an appropriate sense of self-worth. She had to face reality. The food she didn't eat wouldn't go to starving children in India and there was no reason to feel she was stealing it from people who needed it more than she. I helped her to acknowledge that she'd always been a caring and charitable person and that by eating less she could carry on these good deeds during a longer lifetime.

Some clients tell me they were only considered "good" as kids when they cleaned their plates. Notice these thoughts of "naughtiness" if you have them, too. Today, in the here and now, you're being "good" to yourself by *not* overeating, and your parents, whether or not they're still with you, would likely approve of your health-conscious habits. (If they don't, then they probably need—or needed—to learn these techniques, too!)

Lisa, a client to whom I'd just shown these eating techniques, had a troubled look on her face as we waited for her car in the parking lot of the restaurant where we'd dined. When I asked her about it she answered, "I know that I should have finished that dessert!" It had been a strange experience for her to take two or three bites of something she liked and stop eating because she was full. She had a vague sense that she'd cheated herself and this realization was painful. Lisa had been the eldest of five and had always been expected to care for her siblings when her mother was at work or busy pursuing her nursing degree. She resented this but never openly expressed her feelings to anyone. Overeating represented a way of laying claim to her right to do as she chose. Her blatant bingeing, however, had been at the expense of her own health and emotional fulfillment.

Another client, Bev, told me she was struck by a strange realization an hour or two after our meal. She told me that never before in her adult life did she remember finishing a meal without physical pain due to excessive fullness. Eating only to the point of satisfaction had been a unique experience for her. A widow in her sixties, Bev had lost her mother when she was only three and was raised by her father's emotionally distant second wife. Sadly, she'd never known true nurturing. Soon after Bev married she realized that her husband was tyrannical and gave her little freedom in the marriage. Eating had become her only way of nurturing herself, as she tried desperately at every meal to show herself the love she'd lacked in the past. But food wasn't filling her emotional void, and the pain—both physical and psychological—of overeating was taking a toll. Once she realized this we were able to help her mourn her losses and explore new ways to give and get affection. These included volunteer work and more frequent visits with grandchildren.

Jennifer, in her early forties, later spoke of her lingering doubts about whether she'd chosen the most appealing entrée. These concerns had preoccupied her during the meal and even afterward. A successful business executive, Jennifer was in her second marriage and was concerned about not making any more "mistakes" in her personal or professional life. She often felt that "time was running out" and she wouldn't be able to satisfy all her perfectionistic personal and professional goals.

We looked together at the pain this perfectionism was causing her, not only in limiting her enjoyment of food but throughout the rest of her life as well. Once we'd done this work together Jennifer was better able to allow herself a grade of B in a number of activities and to prioritize her enjoyment instead. With respect to her choice of food that evening, we discussed that she could easily return to that restaurant another time to try the entrée she'd rejected. After all, it was only ten minutes from her home, hardly an exotic café in Timbuktu! Adopting a more self-accepting attitude that allowed for trial and error was a life lesson she needed, and not only at the table.

As you practice these techniques you might also experience a feeling of guilt because you stopped at a fullness level of 6.5, rather than at a 6, a 5.5, or a 5. This slight overshooting isn't uncommon since it takes a while to succeed at any new skill. Trying to do this or anything perfectly can cause stress, contribute to depression, and, as discussed earlier, breed bingeing. Instead, next time observe yourself more stringently as you approach satisfaction. Really feel that moment arriving. Note that you experience less urgency before each bite. Your mind may wander away from your meal as you gain a growing awareness that you're eating your food merely because it's there.

Here is some advice that I love, again from Bliss's *Getting Things Done*, interestingly, a book about time management rather than psychotherapy:

> A famous New York psychiatrist, nearing the end of a long and illustrious career . . . said that the most useful concept he had discovered for helping people turn their lives around was what he called his four little words. The first two were *if only*. . . . The antidote is simple: eliminate those two words from your vocabulary. . . . Substitute the words *next time*.[1]

Love it. Like it. Leave it! Yes, you can. And every time you try, you'll do it better—or learn for "next time."

Now we're ready to approach a challenge many novices need help in facing. Have you guessed what it might be? It's their fear of the reaction of others when they don't finish all or most of what's on their plate. Many clients admit to being afraid of the displeasure of the server if they order only soup and a side salad or an appetizer. Others are concerned about being criticized by those at the table and by the restaurant staff if they don't finish everything on their plate.

One solution, of course, is to split a dish with a friend, especially if you expect the serving to be large, as is true in many restaurants. You might also ask if a tempting appetizer is large enough to be satisfying as a meal. Often they come in a "sane-size" rather than a "super-size" portion and are more than adequate as a main course. Another option, when feasible, is to request a doggie bag (which I sometimes do at the very beginning of the meal, assuming the enormity of the offering). There may be rare times, however, when these aren't options.

In these cases, consider your oversensitivity to others' reactions. You'll need to get past this to realize your full potential for enjoying your food and your life. Ask yourself, "What harm will befall me if this server/date/parent/ in-law/spouse disapproves of the way I'm eating this meal?" Most likely the only "harm" to befall you would be your own thoughts and feelings about their response—real or imagined. You might think, "Wouldn't it be awful if they commented on the food I was wasting?" To which you might say to yourself, "So what?"

These concerns may well be linked to your childhood and might stem from missing out on the nurturing you needed. Notice these feelings and be supportive of yourself in order to replenish your store of self-regard right now. Also, it might be helpful to have some stock answers ready for people who disapprove of how sparingly you ate, or more accurately, that you didn't overstuff yourself. Asserting yourself in these situations is an important, self-esteem-building experience. Here are some stock responses, depending on the situation:

- "It's better to throw food out than to throw it in." (If your eating companion is thin.)
- "I was so perfectly satisfied I couldn't eat another bite."
- "What I had was just enough."
- "I'm getting into the habit of eating exactly as much as I'm hungry for and no more." (With an eating companion who's an intimate.)

Feel free to improvise if you wish to respond at all, but keep your answer short and sweet and follow up by changing the subject of conversation.

If people are painfully aware of how much food you're leaving on your plate, they probably have eating issues, too. Those who overeat, drink excessively, or smoke may crave company so as not to feel alone in their addictions. On the other hand, those who are truly enjoying their lives and their food are having too much fun to give a "fig" about what you are or aren't eating!

If you come from a family where others suffered from addictions, or had an addictive need to control you, this aspect of the plan may seem very tough. But asserting yourself with food can be your first step toward asserting yourself elsewhere and may reap far-reaching benefits.

People sometimes stare or comment when they see I've ordered a dessert or picked one from a buffet and have eaten only a few bites. They may act irritated that I've left most of my dessert and they've rapidly finished their own. Often, however, the comments take on a tone of admiration, as in the case of a meal I ate with another therapist, a man who stated that he specialized in weight control and was the president of a large organization of psychotherapists but secretly wanted to lose some weight himself. As he saw the unfinished pie on my plate he said, "You mean you can stop eating when you're full? I wish I could do that!"

If you wish to truly learn these techniques, practice, practice, practice! Your main objective should be to really enjoy your food yet attain peak performance by catching the moment of fullness and taking control.

Remember the **RAFT** concepts—**R**elaxation, **A**wareness, **F**ullness Check, and **T**aking Charge of the Moment—and repeat them to yourself before and during every meal. After a while the steps should come naturally. Just sitting at a table will signal the beginning of your relaxation. You'll automatically start to tune out stress and tune in what's enjoyable, noting your level of pleasure peak and decline as your level of fullness rises. After the meal you'll feel satisfied, healthy, energetic, and light—ready to enjoy the day's or evening's activities. When you know it's the way you'd love to eat for the rest of your life, you know you're doing it right!

You now know the meaning of the third letter in your daily one-minute monitor, "Am I doing what's best for my **SELF**?" It's **L** for **L**oving Your Food.

Before each meal remind yourself to practice these techniques—and enjoy!

6

POINT #4: FLUIDS AND HEALTHY FOODS—LEARN TO LOVE THEM

"Oh, no!" you may be thinking. Here comes the lecture. "In spite of everything I've read before, here's where she's going to tell me that I have to give up all the foods I like and switch to seaweed!" Well, relax. I'm aware that lectures usually do no good. This is a book about loving your food, as well as your life. What part would preaching play in a book about pleasure?

We're continuing on our journey—this time exploring enjoyable new options for satisfying our hunger and appealing to our appetite. Our quest is to land at moderation and balance, discovering new delights along the way. The goal is to make it easy and fun. That's what makes it happen and eventually become a habit.

We'll start by looking at the importance of drinking adequate water. Good hydration is key in helping you embrace pleasurable, nonemotional eating, as well as for overall health. Then we'll explore some healthy eating options. If you're steeling yourself against strict prescriptions, please stop. Most evolved nutritionists today advise a 90 percent healthy, 10 percent fun foods approach. We'll be looking at ways to explore new experiences, tweak our tastes, and enjoy food more.

WATER, WATER EVERYWHERE—BUT DO WE REMEMBER TO DRINK?

Perhaps you've noticed a growing number of people, especially those who look fit and athletic, lugging and chugging their bottles of water everywhere. What do these people know that you may not? Is water really key to controlling your emotional overeating? How much is enough?

We'll address these questions in this chapter, as well as provide practical pointers on how to make good hydration happen for you. While some of this may be familiar, other information may be new, interesting, and even intriguing.

In a chapter titled "Fluids, the Power of Water" from the *American Dietetic Association Complete Food and Nutrition Guide*, Roberta Larson Duyff emphasizes the crucial role hydration plays in our survival.[1] Your body, if you're healthy, is about half water—45 to 75 percent—a requirement for the performance of vital functions essential to life. The amount of water in your body depends on your age, the percentages of muscle in your body, your gender, and other considerations.

Water is required for the performance of almost every bodily function essential to life. It also plays an important role in regulating your body's temperature, because heat changes perspiration from a liquid to a gas, thereby cooling your body. Water provides moisture to many bodily tissues, such as our noses, our mouths, and our eyes. It's also a key component of all of our bodily fluids, including blood, gastric juice, urine, and saliva.

We also rely on water to bring oxygen and nutrients to our cells, as well as to remove waste products. Drinking adequate water serves to keep us regular and maintain softer stools. Water serves to pad our vital organs, including our spinal cord, shielding them from potential injury.

Some people worry about bloating. If we drink an optimum amount of water we can avoid undue water retention. When we don't drink enough water, our body goes into a protective mode and stores as much water as it can to prevent dehydration. If we drink enough water our bodies no longer need to default to this protective mode.

Severe dehydration can cause death. But mild dehydration can leave you feeling fatigued, suffering from a headache, and irritable. Most important, this will threaten your health and lessen your ability to enjoy your life. In addition, if you're home, fatigued and irritable, you may well be prone to overeat.

There are a number of current studies regarding the role of water in weight loss. While the results sometimes conflict, much of the data is intriguing. For example, a recent study out of the University of Michigan indicates that obese people are often less well hydrated, but barring a conclusive cause-and-effect connection, no specific recommendations resulted.[2] Dr. Chang, one of the lead researchers, did conclude that hydration is increasingly being studied as significant in weight loss and that "we often hear recommendations that drinking water is a way to avoid overeating because you may be thirsty rather than hungry."[3] You may have noticed this personally as I have. If so, your observations probably confirm Dr. Chang's professional opinion.

Jane, a single woman in her thirties, couldn't understand why she was gaining weight even though she'd raised her level of exercise. Jane worked out daily at her fitness club for about an hour before dinner, heading there directly from the office. Since she didn't hydrate adequately both before and during exercise, however, she was very thirsty as she sat down to eat (most nutritionists advise eight ounces of water for every fifteen minutes of intense exercise). Unfortunately, she mistook thirst for hunger. Alternating between gulping diet soda and consuming massive amounts of food—very often heavy in carbs, like pasta—she thought she was satisfying hunger, but may only have been assuaging her thirst while she ate. Jane became ensnarled in a syndrome, sadly prevalent in our society, that I'm sure you've seen and may even experience yourself. Whether or not you're afflicted, you may see the symptoms often—at sporting events, movie theaters, even perhaps in your home.

I've named it the "munch 'n' gulp"—a combo of drinking a beverage (often beer or something sweet) along with a salty food—like chips, buffalo wings, popcorn, or nuts—all in an attempt to disassociate from stress, an escape to a world of our own. The salty food sets up the need for fluid, and the tasty fluid momentarily quenches that thirst in a way that assures us that, yes, we can satisfy our needs.

This is a misguided attempt at stress management. It's a desperate, though momentarily enjoyable, attempt at distraction and disconnecting from our existing reality, which when done at full speed, with copious amounts of food and drink, can result in the consumption of a lot of calories. Have you ever eaten a large popcorn, heavily buttered and salted, at a movie theater and later wondered why?

One approach to controlling the munch 'n' gulp syndrome is good hydration. If you aren't thirsty, you're less likely to engage in the practice often, and if so, you may do so in moderation or better still (!) in miniature. For example, going to a movie or sporting event well hydrated makes it easier to drink a small portion of soda or to order a kid-size or senior-size bag of popcorn, bowl of chips, or whatever. Incidentally, you don't have to be a child to order kid-size meals at movies, fast-food chains, or almost anywhere. (Anyone might have a five-year-old in the car or at home!) Feed your "inner child" for a healthier you.

I suggest you replace "munch 'n' gulp" with "sip and savor." Take small sips of your beverage—you aren't thirsty so you don't need to gulp—with small bites, say, one piece of popcorn at a time, rather than whole handfuls. Pretend you're a connoisseur of whatever you're eating, a professional popcorn taster, perhaps. Because your job is to rate the color, texture, and taste of the offerings at various venues, your responsibility is to note what renders each piece of popped corn unique. Be a gourmet. Replacing mindless snacking with a more sensual, savoring approach will maximize your pleasure, while reducing the amount you eat.

I do this myself. Because I've learned to reduce and refine this behavior I actually enjoy it more. Several times, attending a movie solo that coincided with lunch or dinnertime, I've ordered a kid-size popcorn combo, topped it lightly with butter, and savored it throughout the flick. Following it with a piece of fruit for dessert, I've called it lunch— or dinner. I'm not a purist. Evolving past emotional overeating means being the best we can realistically be. (Incidentally, if the movie isn't interesting after you're finished your popcorn, you may be watching the wrong flicks. Check out the reviews in advance next time. Ebert.com is my favorite, but find your own. If you read a few reviewers regularly, you'll soon spot who's in sync with your preferences. Honor yourself, your time, and treat yourself well in every way.)

Returning to hydration, we are still left with the big question about water. *How much is enough?* There's currently some controversy. The standard thinking from nutritionists and exercise physiologists used to be to drink at least one ounce for every two pounds of body weight—or approximately 70 ounces of water for a 140-pound woman. Many of us might feel that's hard to do. But since many other fluids count, along with fluid-filled foods (lettuce is 90 percent water!), the task is less daunting. Broth-based soups are also a wonderful option. But beware of what comes with some of those fluids. Fruit juices, sodas, and alcoholic beverages may carry many calories, while other drinks such as coffee, tea, and colas come with caffeine, a diuretic that can dehydrate.

Jodi Stookey, a nutritional epidemiologist and hydration researcher at the Children's Hospital Oakland Research Institute, conducted a study concluding that drinking at least four glasses of water a day aided weight loss: "Water can actually help promote weight loss in many ways. By substituting water for sugary beverages or juice, you've removed calories and carbohydrates. Then, if you have enough water, you can start seeing more efficient insulin pathways and an acceleration of fat burning."[4]

There are many different sources of water, some surprising. According to Carroll A. Lutz and Karen Rutherford Przytulski, authors of *Nutrition & Diet Therapy: Evidence-Based Applications*,

> We obtain 4 cups of water per day in foods. Some foods that are solids also have a high water content: a head of lettuce is 96 percent water, celery is 95 percent water, and raw carrots are 88 percent water. Other foods that contain a large percentage of water include apples (84 percent), grapes (81 percent), bananas (74 percent), hard-cooked eggs (75 percent), drained tuna (61 percent), and chicken breast or thigh (52 percent). Whole wheat bread is 38 percent water: its water content drops to 29 percent when the bread is toasted.[5]

This gives new meaning to "water, water everywhere," doesn't it? And it also makes what's often described as an ideal goal of eight glasses a day seem more doable.

Many experts say that there is no specific one-size-fits-all to the question, "How much?" The optimum amount depends on your size, age, level of activity, and the temperature. Since this book is about improvement, not perfection, I can only advise you to drink as much as feels right and keeps your urine light (no darker than pale yellow), and if you're active, to try to drink more.

Try to avoid an all-or-nothing, do-or-die, dieter's mind-set. One woman I spoke with, in her sixties, who has struggled with food and weight for decades said, "When I attended meetings of [a popular dieting group] I drank eight glasses of water a day. But now I drink nothing, unless I'm exercising outside in the heat."

Now that you know that more is better, within reason, you may be asking, "How?" Start by trying to have a glass of water prior to each meal. If you drink it with minimal ice, as is often customary in Europe and other parts of the world, it's easier to consume. Carrying a water bottle so that water is always available will also help visually prompt you, something we'll discuss more later.

If you crave a sugary beverage, you might try to dilute it with ice and order some water, too. You may be surprised that several sips of the sugary stuff are all you really want. If weight is an issue and you like a cocktail or two at dinner, you'd do best to cut it down. Drinking water alongside your alcoholic beverage or ordering water after only one cocktail at a party are two strategies clients have tried (reporting back, with relief, that they weren't seen as "party poopers"!).

If you're upping water intake, frequent urination may pose an issue, especially if you're female, gave birth naturally, or are over forty. Allow yourself to go to the bathroom whenever necessary—since females, embarrassed about excusing themselves, are more susceptible to bladder issues. If you're engaging in active sports or aerobic classes, you may choose to wear a pad to prevent accidents. It's a small price to pay to achieve better health.

FOOD, GLORIOUS FOOD

Since I've trained as a psychotherapist, not a nutritionist, I've written this book to help you better understand how and why you eat, rather than what. But I'd like us all to embrace an awareness of how our food choices feel. It's dismaying that so many of us are stuck in the rut of a boring, overly processed, carb-laden diet. It's aptly referred to as SAD (standard American diet). SAD, inactivity, and the ubiquity of super-size rather than sane-size portions raised the number of overweight Americans to record levels—over 70 percent at this writing.

How does this affect your efforts to end your emotional overeating? Filling up first on healthy, fluid-filled foods allows you to gain control of intake more easily. If weight is an issue, eating the more calorie-intense items later in the meal may make them less compelling. Also, when you're truly satisfied, snacking afterward is a less appealing option. Finally, eating well and being healthier feels better. This adds to our enthusiasm for doing other good things for ourselves, like exercising. It's a feedback loop leading onward and upward throughout the synergistic aspects of this plan.

Feeling better and less stressed also helps us make good choices. A 2015 study published in *Neuron* tested whether greater perceived stress influenced the food choices made by participants. The researchers recruited fifty-one men who stated that they were trying to make healthier food choices. Half were given the potentially stressful task of placing their hands in icy water, which raised their cortisol levels and indicated that it caused them stress. Subsequently, they were shown foods on computer screens, paired so that half were healthy and half could be categorized as "junk." Those who experienced the most stress made the least healthy choices, opting for short-term taste intensity rather than long-term healthful objectives.[6]

So keep checking in to see how you feel, managing your stress by gently responding to pain-producing thoughts and exercising often— the latter being one of the main forms of stress reduction advised by the study's authors.

By now you should be ready to start planning some healthier choices. But which foods really are the healthiest? In the face of data that often conflicts, even the acclaimed experts rarely come to a consensus.

In his entertaining and informative *If Our Bodies Could Talk*, James Hamblin, MD, describes a 2015 meeting that was held for twenty-five of the most renowned nutritionists in the world. Although noting a great deal of discord among them, he did write this:

> Every one of the twenty-five scientists in the room did agree that people should eat vegetables. And fruits, nuts, seeds, and legumes. They all agreed that this should be the basis of everyone's diet. There should be variety, and there should not be excessive "processing" of the foods. The devil was in how to say this. They stayed until midnight that day in Boston, trying to figure it out.[7]

You may be thinking that a plant-based diet, even a varied version that affords for other food groups, might be boring. But when we tweak our choices, we often acquire new tastes.

The other day I visited a local farm-to-table eatery. I remembered that their vegetable plate was amazing and that it changed daily according to availability. I wasn't disappointed. At first glance the dish looked like a work of art, arrayed with vivid colors, the soft green of an avocado sauce gracefully swirling on the border of the square white plate. The cauliflower, cooked just right—slightly al dente—was sumptuous, as was the broccoli, a dark robust green. The corn was amazing. It was vividly yellow, sweet, and lightly accented by some vibrant red peppers. I first drank a glass of water, and then had an iced tea on the side. The meal was so satisfying and filling that I took home almost half to serve with dinner later.

My conversation with the waiter revealed I'm not alone in favoring the venue. A world-renowned former basketball star (maybe the best known of all time), a current leading golfer, and a top ten tennis star are all among its clientele. What convincing confirmation that I was doing what's best for my body!

Along the same lines, in 2015 a panel of physicians, dieticians, and nutritionists, which included input from experts at New York–Presbyterian Hospital and the John Hopkins Weight Management Center, reported to *U.S. News & World Report* that their favorite diet was the DASH diet, similar in many ways to the Mediterranean diet.[8] It scored high in many categories including "safety," "nutrition," and "easy to follow." The diet was originally designed to lower blood pressure, and includes a mix of whole grains, lean protein, fruits, and vegetables. It suggests that red meats, sweets, and salt be eaten less often.

Although the DASH diet was named overall "best" by the magazine, the U.S. government panel that put together the 2015 Dietary Guidelines for Americans gave the Mediterranean diet as an example of the healthiest way to eat. Which is preferable? Kathy McManus, director of the Department of Nutrition at Harvard-affiliated Brigham and Women's Hospital, recommends both to patients.[9]

The DASH diet is more prescriptive, giving exact numbers of servings of each of the food groups. Daily: whole grains, 7–8; vegetables, 4–5; fruits, 4–5; dairy, low fat, or nonfat, 2–3; lean meats, poultry, fish, 2 or fewer. Weekly: nuts, seeds, dry beans, 4–5; fats and oils, 2–3; sweets, 5.

The Mediterranean, on the other hand, is based on a pyramid, with a large lower level of whole grains, fruits, seeds, olive oil, beans, nuts, legumes—on which every meal is to be based; topped by fish or seafood—to be eaten at least twice a week; then poultry, eggs, yogurt, cheese—to be eaten in moderate portions during the week; meats and sweets—to be eaten less often; and wine—which can be drunk in moderation.

Does this sound doable? Does it seem potentially pleasurable? Patterns you might like to move toward practicing? To me it does. Though I've been moving in this direction for a while, this information only encourages me to continue exploring and enjoying new food options along the way.

So keep your ears open. Read up. Explore what may be best, easiest, and most fun for you. Most of all, be open to tweaking old patterns and trying new possibilities.

What other tips might be helpful?

For many years, my husband and I have chosen to start many of our meals with soup (for me, usually broth based) and/or a salad. We find it a pleasurable way to earn some brownie points for fruits and veggies, as well as to feel fuller.

Research has shown that starting with soup can also aid in weight control. Along with many other excellent suggestions on filling up with fluids and less energy dense foods, Barbara Rolls, coauthor of *The Volumetrics Weight-Control Plan: Feel Full on Fewer Calories*, writes, "Soup evokes satiety in just about every way we know a food can."[10] So start your meal with soup, a salad, or both. It's a healthy way to be on your way to satiation.

But this leaves us facing still another challenge—the size of the portion on your plate. It's tough to track your trek toward fullness when your baggage is a portion that's much larger than you need. We're all familiar with the mega sizes of much of the fare we're offered—sixteen-ounce sodas and other monstrously large fast-food options, just to name a few. On the other hand, if we travel, especially abroad, we may be pleasantly surprised to see that portions are often sane-size rather than super-size.

Even within America, there are variations. New Orleans, a town I adore, does celebrate overindulgence. Visiting recently, I passed through a doorway topped by a sign touting "The Best Pralines in New

Orleans." Given that it was a sultry summer day, I wandered toward the ice cream, ordering one praline-flavored scoop on a cone. The proprietor, a congenial, middle-aged man, looked puzzled. "Only one scoop?" he questioned, and paused, his head cocked to the side in quandary. "Yes," I answered, smiling. "Portion control." To which he laughed, loudly retorting, "What the hell is that?" We both were chuckling as I left, my cone in hand, dripping deliciously.

Don't let others deter you, playfully or not. Order small, sane-size portions that you savor sensuously until stopping at satisfaction. You deserve your pleasure *and* your health.

Unfortunately, there are far more forces opposed to our efforts to moderate the amount we eat. It's corporate America. Every day, behind closed doors, conspirators converge to devise new, more nefarious methods to entice you to overeat. Let's take a peek at how this happens. *The End of Overeating: Taking Control of the Insatiable American Appetite*, by David A. Kessler, MD, a former FDA commissioner who took on the tobacco industry, bares the behind-the-scenes efforts of the food industry to bring us to the "bliss point":

> Most of us have what's called a "bliss point"—the point at which we get the most pleasure from sugar, fat, or salt. Scientists depict this as an inverted U-shaped curve: As more sugar is added, food becomes more pleasurable until we reach the bliss point at the top of the curve, and then the pleasure experience drops off. . . . But when the mix is right, food becomes more stimulating. Eating foods high in sugar, fat, and salt makes us eat *more* [emphasis his] foods high in sugar, fat, and salt. We see this clearly both in animal and human research. [11]

Does any of this hit home? Think about cheesecake, buffalo wings, chocolate chip cookies, and that single scoop of praline ice cream I ordered! That's why I advise to limit the amounts of these you keep on hand. If I really want a chocolate chip cookie, I'll buy one and only one that's *great*. For me it's a treat from a local health food eatery that offers an individual, all natural, sane-size version, which I savor at home with a glass of nonfat milk.

Often it's hard to visualize exactly how much a sane-size serving might be. Happily, there are guidelines that are always available. What are they? Our hands. [12] Let's illustrate; see figure 6.1.

There are two ways to make use of this information. You can dole out your own sane servings, rather than super-size ones. It's easier to remember what's right for your body if you've got a guide that's always on hand (literally and figuratively!). (See Figure 6.1.) Second, these standards, emblazoned in your memory, enable you to view the extent to which you're being overserved when eating out. Whenever this occurs I either offer to share, or request a doggie bag as soon as possible (another good reason to adopt a pup as your extra protein will delight your dog). I then take charge, by leaving an appropriately sized serving on my plate, while allotting the rest to the to-go container.

If the discussion so far has been intriguing, even appealing, start to make small changes and see how they feel. If you're eating a great deal of carbs, consider cutting one overly processed carb a day (think white bread or store-bought cookies) and replacing it with a plant-based food instead.

Neither carbs nor fats per se, as once thought, are enemies in our efforts to eat healthier. But what exactly are carbs? The answer itself is complex (!) but worth understanding. As we see in the *American Medical Association Complete Guide to Prevention and Wellness,*

> Simple and complex sugars, starches, and fiber from plant foods are the main component of carbohydrates. Carbs come in two types: simple and complex. Simple carbs are sugars, including the sugar found in fruit (fructose), the milk sugar (lactose), and the white sugar in your sugar bowl (sucrose). Simple carbs taste sweet and are easy to digest. However, because they are so easily digestible, they can cause a sudden rise in blood sugar (glucose) levels—something a person with diabetes (or prediabetes) has to avoid.
>
> Foods made from simple carbohydrates of starches, such as white bread, white rice, or white pasta, have been highly refined. This means that the fiber-rich outer bran and nourishing inner germ of the grain have been removed, leaving only the vitamin-and-mineral-poor inside of the seed. This starchy leftover is digested quickly and speeds to the bloodstream, where it can sharply elevate blood sugar. For this reason, doctors tell people who already have elevated blood sugar to limit their intake of foods containing simple sugars.
>
> Complex carbs, on the other hand, get absorbed into the bloodstream slowly. Because foods containing complex carbs—such as whole-grain breads, brown rice, cooked dried beans, and vegetables—take a longer time to digest, they don't reach the bloodstream

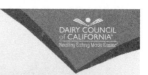

Serving-Size Chart

FOOD	SYMBOL	COMPARISON	SERVING SIZE
Dairy: Milk, Yogurt, Cheese			
Cheese (string cheese)		Pointer finger	1½ ounces
Milk and yogurt (glass of milk)		One fist	1 cup
Vegetables			
Cooked carrots		One fist	1 cup
Salad (bowl of salad)		Two fists	2 cups
Fruits			
Apple		One fist	1 medium
Canned peaches		One fist	1 cup
Grains: Breads, Cereals, Pasta			
Dry cereal (bowl of cereal)		One fist	1 cup
Noodles, rice, oatmeal (bowl of noodles)		Handful	½ cup
Slice of whole-wheat bread		Flat hand	1 slice
Protein: Meat, Beans, Nuts			
Chicken, beef, fish, pork (chicken breast)		Palm	3 ounces
Peanut butter (spoon of peanut butter)		Thumb	1 tablespoon

HealthyEating.org

Figure 6.1.   Serving-Size Chart (Courtesy of the Dairy Council of California, HealthyEating.org)

all at once. Another benefit: these foods contain a lot more vitamins, minerals, and other nutrients than simple carbs.[13]

Although the answer wasn't simple, it was hopefully intriguing and sufficiently enticing that you're tempted to expand your daily choices to include more complex carbs. String beans, for example, had never been my favorite food. But a local Asian buffet serves them al dente, grilled in olive oil and garlic, with the perfect seasoning to make their flavor pop. Whenever I'm there I love to fill up on veggies, relegating all other options, even their ice cream, lower on my list of preferences.

How about fats? Many of us believe that low-fat options are always optimal, but they may be high in calories, and as with carbs, all fats are not created equally nor do they impact our bodies in the same way.

In a posting from Harvard Health Publishing, "The Truth about Fats: The Good, the Bad, and the In-Between" (August 22, 2017), some of the controversy on this subject is clarified. At one point all fats were considered harmful, but because fat is vital for the proper functioning of our bodies—for the building of cells, blood clotting, inflammation, and muscle usage—fats have been classified into categories. The best fats are monounsaturated and polyunsaturated: olive oil, peanut oil, canola oil, avocados, and most nuts. Polyunsaturated fats, which lessen our LDL cholesterol and lower triglycerides, and are also beneficial, can be found in salmon, mackerel, sardines, flaxseeds, walnuts, canola oil, and unhydrogenated soybean oil. Less beneficial, so it's suggested that we keep them to less than 10 percent of our daily caloric intake, are saturated fats, derived from red meat, whole milk, cheese, coconut oils, and many commercially made cakes and cookies. The most harmful are known as trans fats, which were commonly found in french fries and store-bought cookies and pastries, but due to health concerns are fortunately becoming less common.[14]

You can learn more from other reputable institutions and government sources, such as choosemyplate.gov, the Weight-control Information Network (WIN), the National Institutes of Health (NIH), and the CDC, which are only a finger's touch away on your cell phone or PC—so read up.

As you learn more about how the best foods help your body, healthy choices will become more appealing. Why is it important to do this? The coercion to eat unhealthy foods is constant. We're barraged by images of energy-dense foodstuffs, often engineered to be "blissfully" high in sugar, fat, and salt. How can we counteract this?

Try to create your own tricks to remember to eat what's good for you but also tastes good. Explore your supermarket; keep to the outer reaches where items are of the whole-foods variety and less processed. In your fridge at home, keep fruit, an ideal snack, at eye level. Try to keep vegetables there as well—a visual cue to use them before they spoil. (Location, location, and location!)

Keep abreast of foods that may be most beneficial. Sign up (via email or snail mail) for newsletters (like the ones mentioned here), magazines, pamphlets, and other materials produced to promote your health and well-being. Keep the information where it's visible and do whatever you can to make sure it influences your shopping list.

Some foods recently showcased in the *Nutrition Action Healthletter*, published by the nonprofit Center for Science in the Public Interest, are

- Sweet potatoes—rich in carotenoids, and a moderate source of Vitamin C, potassium and fiber.
- Mangoes—one cupful provides a day's requirements of vitamin C, a third of a day's vitamin A, potassium, and three grams of fiber.
- Unsweetened Greek yogurt—a good source of protein, especially tasty with fresh fruit, such as bananas, which will add a dollop of potassium.
- Broccoli—full of vitamin C, carotenoids, vitamin K, and folic acid.
- Wild salmon—contains omega-3 fats, which may lessen the risk of heart disease, depression, diabetes, and more.
- Watermelon—contains one-third of a day's vitamins A and C requirements, plus potassium and lycopene.
- Butternut squash—good source of vitamins A and C and fiber.
- Oatmeal.
- Garbanzo beans.
- Leafy greens—dense with vitamins like A, C, and K; folate; potassium; magnesium; calcium; iron; and fiber. If you haven't tried kale you may be pleasantly surprised by its subtle, fresh taste and fun, crunchy texture.[15]

Keep an open mind, exploring, experimenting with new options, trying new tastes and treats, or appreciating familiar flavors even more. Sounds like an adventure, doesn't it?

You now know the meaning of the last letter in **SELF**—learning to love **F**luids and healthy **F**oods. Since SAD can be boring, why not break free and try what's not only better for you but more fun?! I hope you will.

7

POINT #5: EVENING EATING—"ARE YOU A 'LIGHT' EATER?"

Anyone who has ever tried to lose weight or keep weight off realizes that evening can be the make or break time of day in terms of permanent success.

Consider this. In my community there currently is a radio-based advertising campaign touting the effectiveness of a weight loss formula that I will refer to as the Weight Loss Answer. This liquid, taken at bedtime, is to be consumed on an empty stomach. The purchaser is told not to eat or drink anything for three hours prior to drinking the "miracle product," which will melt pounds away regardless of whatever is eaten during the day. The radio announcer who is advocating this product sounds somewhat manic (a side effect of the product or the promotional fee?) and swears that he has shed over twenty pounds in about six months.

And now I'm going to tell you a money-saving secret. If you keep a journal of everything you eat all day, and are especially scrupulous about writing everything you eat in the evening, chances are that 20 to 30 percent of your day's calories are consumed not in the day, but at night! By deducting most, if not all, of the calories ingested in the evening, you can probably make your own "miracle," and keep your hard-earned money.

Let's do the math. Let's say you eat six chocolate chip cookies with a glass of milk while watching television. Later on, as you read a book, you slowly suck on a low-fat Popsicle. Somewhat later, while watching more TV and speaking on the phone, you munch somewhat mindlessly on several small bowls of popcorn with a glass of orange juice on the side. If this scenario sounds too familiar to acknowledge, don't be afraid to admit it, because I have snacked exactly in this manner myself!

Six chocolate chip cookies at 50 calories per cookie	300 calories
One cup low-fat milk	90 calories
Low-fat Popsicle	70 calories
One serving popcorn	150 calories
One eight-ounce glass orange juice	110 calories

Have you done the addition? This one night of "light" snacking "weighs in" at a total of 720 calories. All it takes is 3,500 additional calories a week, or 500 per day, to result in a gain of one pound of weight per week. Eliminating most, but not necessarily all, of these tasty treats means four pounds less per month for most of us, or twelve pounds in three months, and a whopping forty-eight pounds in a year. That's not even counting the extra calories you're now expending because you exercise for thirty minutes most days!

Aside from the weight loss benefits of controlling evening eating, there is even more good news. Reflux, often referred to as heartburn or indigestion, is a common condition affecting as many as one in five Americans at least once per week.[1] Avoiding eating for three hours prior to bedtime is one way to lessen or eliminate the symptoms of this annoying ailment.

Excessive evening eating is a common downfall of those who would love to be slim, yet rarely, if ever, succeed. The syndrome of what I call "thief in the night noshing" is rampant. This "crime" is so common that probably someone you know falls on the Most Wanted list. What does the modus operandi look like? First, the burglar hurries into the kitchen, hastily scanning the crime scene in an attempt to avoid detection. Then, he or she cases the joint for the stash of "illegal" goodies—cake, cookies, or ice cream, let's say. The culprit usually eats swiftly while standing up, barely tasting and hardly enjoying the large quantities of food consumed, ready for a quick getaway in case anyone else should arrive.

If you recognize yourself in this scenario, you may feel frustrated. (And yes, in the past I was guilty myself.) All too often clients report,

"I've been good all day, loving my food, but at night I eat and eat and just can't stop." So what's the solution to this all-too-common "crime"?

The clues, and that's where much of the solution exists, are revealed well before the evening begins. You need to eat enough throughout the day, drink enough water, and exercise sufficiently so that you enter the evening feeling relatively satisfied, tired, and relaxed. Eat three well-balanced meals and don't neglect dinner, even if you live alone or dine alone. Many people find it hard to be self-nurturing in this way. They can find time to cook for their families, or their friends, but not, unfortunately, for themselves.

I am reminded of a story about a man who was knocking at St. Peter's gate and was told, "Come on in. You're just in time for dinner. Here's a telescope so that you can keep yourself entertained looking down below while you wait for your meal." At that point, St. Peter excuses himself and the new arrival looks down below. To his surprise everyone there is dining on shrimp cocktail, then consommé, a salad, filet mignon, and at the end a chocolate mousse for dessert. Finally, St. Peter returns, bearing a TV dinner on a tray. "What?" asks the newcomer. "How come all of them down there are eating a five-course gourmet dinner and I'm eating this?" "Cook just for one?" responds St. Peter.

There's truth in this joke, which is why so many of my single friends in Manhattan used to laugh at that story. We all have the tendency to neglect our own nutrition and pleasure when eating alone. Remind yourself that you deserve to treat yourself well in all ways and at all times. Pick up easy to prepare foods that you can eat and enjoy if you arrive home late and tired. Set the table. Buy yourself flowers. Sit down, relax, and dine.

If you are able to, treat yourself on occasion to a meal in a restaurant, allowing yourself to love not only the food but the solitude as well. Using the eating techniques we outlined earlier, you can create a relaxing mood and be assured that you will have a congenial companion.

One of my favorite writers was M. F. K. Fisher, an unforgettable woman who may have been the first famous foodie of the modern era. Her love of food was matched by an incomparably independent attitude, something rather novel in the early twentieth century. In the late 1930s, voyaging alone during a difficult time in her marriage, she wrote,

I discovered, there on the staidly luxurious Dutch liner, that I could be very firm with pursers and stewards and such. I could have a table assigned to me in any part of the dining room I wanted, and best of all I could have that table to myself. I needed no longer be put with officers or predatory passengers, just because I was under ninety and predominantly female. It would never again matter to me that the purser would look oddly at me for my requests, and that people stared and whispered when I walked alone to my table; I had what I needed to bolster my own loneliness, a sense of strength.

And once seated I could eat what I wanted and drink what I wanted. I could spend all the time I needed over a piece of *pâté*, truly to savor its uncountable tastes; I could make a whole meal of little lettuce hearts and buttermilk, or ask for frogs legs *provençale* and *pêches* Victoria—and get them.

And if I felt like it, I could invite another passenger to dine with me, and order an intelligent thoughtful meal, to please the chef and the wine steward. That was enjoyable occasionally, but in general I preferred to eat by myself, slowly, voluptuously and with an independence that heartened me against the coldness of my cabin and my thoughts.[2]

Savor your dinner, no matter where or with whom you dine. Value, as did Fisher, your ability to eat "voluptuously," whether with others or alone. Entertain your most pleasant thoughts, similarly to the way you'd select the most enjoyable topics of conversation if you were out with a friend. Treat yourself with respect and kindness.

Also consider the scenario that ensues after dinner. You've eaten and yet you still have the desire for something sweet. Occasionally, allow yourself one small treat to savor early in the evening. It doesn't have to be an executive decision that you arrive at by 9 a.m., but as evening rolls around, and by the time that dinner's over, you might begin to think about which small sweet will bring you the most pleasure. A pleasant preoccupation, isn't it?

The classic musical *A Chorus Line* featured a knockout number called "One Singular Sensation." Likewise, choosing only one small singular sensation of a snack will help you feel more like the singular sensation you are, because when you eat less in the evening, you'll almost immediately feel lighter, more energetic, and generally better about yourself the next day.

When indulging in that mini-snack, be sure to apply the same techniques we used in chapter 5, "Love Your Food." Let's say, for example, that it's a small, fun-size Snickers bar, which you're having as you sip a glass of low-fat milk. Unwrap the candy bar. Look at it. Notice the wave-like swirls of milk chocolate covering the top of the bar. Hold it in your hand and sniff it, savoring the sensuous pleasure it promises. Take a bite. What do you notice? You may taste an intriguing blend of chocolate and nut-like flavors that combine and intermittently compete. Perhaps you especially enjoy the texture of the bar as you bite into it, firm yet forgiving enough to melt slowly in your mouth as you chew. The smooth chocolate, somewhat grittier nougat, creamy caramel, and crunchy nuts present a medley of tastes and textures. You might, in addition, notice a rather salty taste, which beckons you to eat more—perhaps more than you'd otherwise really want. Take an occasional sip of milk, if you choose, as you savor your snack.

What memories does this treat bring back for you? Does it remind you of childhood, special children's parties, or Halloween? Let the sensations take you back to a time that felt safe, secure, and pleasant. There is a very pleasant memory that is evoked for me when I eat a Snickers bar. I remember a neighbor's home in our suburban community where I used to trick or treat as a child. She had set up a mini-size candy counter and invited each child who entered to choose his or her favorite confection. Thinking back on that wondrous surprise brings me tremendous pleasure—a carefree, childlike joy. So take a while to savor your snack, enjoying the sight, scent, taste, and texture of it, as well as the memories.

The more enjoyment you derive from your snack, the better. The realization that you can choose to do so as much as once a day (although as time goes by you may choose to lessen that to once or twice a week) will cut into your craving for excessive amounts of these foods at other times. But keep in mind that since your snack of choice may well have been engineered with the bliss factor in mind, you may not want to keep much of it on hand. Anything built to sabotage your sense of satiation isn't something to keep available in large quantities—especially while you're new to these techniques.

As time goes on you may find that your taste for treats changes. Lately I've found that fresh-cut fruits are often more appealing than the bliss-factored foods I formerly used to crave. I love the different colors, shapes, and tastes. The cheery cherry-toned sweetness of watermelon reminds me of a summer's day up north and the long-awaited warmth and relaxation of that season, including, for us kids, time off from school!

Give your preferences the chance to change and evolve. You may be amazed at how satisfying other options can be when you don't stereotype your tastes to typical dessert-type fare.

That is your first strategy toward handling evening eating. You may have noticed that I advised that you eat your treat early in the evening, if at all. The second strategy may be far more challenging, but it's one of the most healthful to follow each day. Choose a cutoff time, preferably three and a half to four hours prior to your bedtime, after which you do not eat. Does that seem hard if not impossible to do? What you now need to do is analyze how you spend your time in the evening.

Jane, a married woman whose husband often came home two or three hours later than she did, told me that she liked to read in the evening, but it was very hard for her to read without munching or sucking on a snack. Together we looked at what she was reading and whether it really intrigued her. The answer was a definite no. When Jane was reading a really riveting novel, time flew by and she preferred to do nothing else but envelop herself in the storyline. The mindless, tasteless stuffing that she did when she was reading something boring was an attempt to distract herself from stressful thoughts and feelings, in a way that the book, alone, failed to do.

So start to critique the books you're reading (making sure that they're great, not just good), the television shows you're watching, and the movies you're attending or streaming. If the movie seems dull after you've finished your popcorn, it probably wasn't worth watching in the first place.

If your evenings seem endless, you may need to spice them up with enjoyable, out of home activities, if not every evening, then at least once or twice per week to break the monotony. Perhaps a sport you enjoy in the daytime such as tennis, racquetball, squash, or even skiing could be engaged in at night.

Search the internet or check out a local community paper to find out if anything of interest is happening. Try that class you'd been considering to learn something new or improve an existing skill. Have you always wanted to play an instrument? Why not do it now? There's a special pleasure in learning a new skill as an adult, especially if we allow ourselves to do it for pleasure rather than demanding a perfect performance.

Snacking could be a wake-up call that you need to live your life more fully. If, in spite of these suggestions, you find yourself staring at the refrigerator, what you're seeking is probably not food. Ask yourself what it might be—friendship, stimulation, love? Once you recognize what you're seeking you can take positive steps to make that happen for yourself.

If this rings true for you, walk from the refrigerator to a table, take a piece of paper, and try to get in touch with what you're seeking. Begin by writing down what you're feeling at the moment and see where that takes you. If you do get a specific sense of some way in which you'd like to change your life, try to think of at least one small step you could take that would give you a sense that you're moving your life in that direction, and if possible, do it within the next day. Don't stare out at the fridge; look inside yourself for answers instead!

If the urge to overeat persists, ask yourself if some residue from the day or early evening is upsetting you. Is there a disturbing feeling that you feel desperate to escape? Let's look again at our working definition of compulsive overeating, which you may remember from chapter 1:

Emotional overeating can be defined as eating neither for enjoyment nor for the satisfaction of hunger, but in a desperate attempt to escape painful thoughts and feelings.

Rather than trying to escape those thoughts and feelings, face them and find a way to comfort yourself in your pain. Has someone hurt you? Are you feeling angry? Use the awareness-building techniques we discussed earlier to discover your feelings and the cognitions that are causing them. Then respond in a logical, self-loving way to any pain-producing thoughts. For example, perhaps someone has done something to hurt you and you catch yourself thinking, "I shouldn't feel this way." One possible response might be, "But I do feel this way and it's natural. Now what can I do in the future to protect myself from similar pain?"

Melissa, a client in her forties, was tempted to binge due to anger. Although it took a while for her to realize what she was experiencing, she allowed her urge to binge to be the "awareness alarm" that she was upset. She knew she had several options, including two of which we had discussed. One option was to call a comforting friend. But she chose the other option, which was potentially more therapeutic because it's more practical on a permanent basis. She spoke to herself and answered herself as if she were that friend. Before long she came to not only the source of her pain, but also the solution, the biggest bonanza of facing rather than fleeing our hidden frustrations.

Melissa had recently met a woman who was a colleague and, in spite of initial doubts, she had decided to pursue a friendship. But the colleague almost immediately started to take advantage of her, first sticking her with a dinner tab, then requesting help on a very time-consuming project, and finally creating dissention between her and other coworkers. When Melissa walked away from the refrigerator and faced her thoughts and feelings she came to an important realization. She was angry not only with her newfound "friend," but she was even angrier with herself for ignoring her initial instincts that this person would cause her pain. On further reflection, however, she realized that there was little she could have done to prevent the future events once she sensed the impending problem. But at present, there was action she could take. Once she came up with a game plan to lessen further damage from this disturbed individual—by gradually diminishing contact in a tactful, subtle way—she immediately felt better. When Melissa stopped blaming herself and others, she could comfort herself and protect herself from further abuse.

Melissa came from a family where she had been taught to sacrifice herself for others and had a mother who did so at almost any cost. As Melissa analyzed this further, she was able to see that her former family "script" sometimes served to initially blind her to people who took undue advantage. This was an important and helpful realization. It helped her to be on the watch for people who might target her as an easy mark for furthering their own selfish needs. By facing rather than fleeing her uncomfortable thoughts and feelings, Melissa found not only comfort, but also a way to better control her future.

As you may have noticed the word *awareness* keeps popping up throughout this book. Indeed, the importance of awareness when working on any type of behavior change cannot be overstated. Only by becoming acutely aware of the steps leading to our present behavior will we be able to change our patterns and develop new habits. Let's analyze evening eating by placing you on your doorstep, about to walk into your home after a typical day. Unfortunately, for most adults in our current high tech society there will be only two activities on the agenda—screen-watching and eating—so the only questions they will ponder will be "How much?" and "What?"

If that's the case with you, it's time to start thinking seriously about expanding your repertoire and becoming more productive and versatile during the last part of your day. There are emotional dangers to too much screen time. I'm hearing it so often from my clients that I've decided to give it a name—social media–induced stress disorder—SMSD.

Here's how it sounds.

"I can't believe I saw my ex-husband on vacation with my former best friend on Instagram! Nothing could get me more upset!"

"How come all these other people are doing the apps and internet start-ups I'd like to launch? It irks me to no end to see them succeeding when I haven't even begun!"

"There he was, my former boyfriend, with this gorgeous girl in a bikini, when all I can wear is a one-piece or a tankini. Just looking at it made me crave a huge ice cream sundae!"

As social media becomes increasingly more pervasive I hear more and more of these statements in psychotherapy sessions. They call to mind a birthday card I saw on sale in Grand Central Station several years ago, which read, "Happy Birthday—May your day be as great as everyone else's appears to be on Facebook!"

If you believe the hype that's posted on Facebook, Instagram, and Twitter you're at heightened risk for SMSD. Keep in mind that what you'll see on social media almost never includes the anguish that's so real when our aspirations do miss the mark. We don't read about interviews that didn't result in an offer, only that our friends have a new and prestigious position. No one posts about a wrecked romance, but we do see a photo of a flashy new flame. The trip that may have been a nightmare appears to be a dream vacation when posted. If we're prone to believe that others have it all—perfect lives, looks, and lovers—social media offers innumerable excuses to make those myths seem true.

This is especially perilous for those of us prone to emotional overeating. Why? Because all of this hype when contrasted with ourselves—as living, struggling, striving, growing, changing, adjusting, and aging human beings—emphasizes a reality that inevitably falls short of an unattainable fantasy of perfection. If we think perfection is possible, then falling short of that utopian standard means somehow we're to blame. That's an awful feeling, and those of us with the tendency to turn to a substance to self-soothe—including food—will be at heightened risk.

When I was single and living in Manhattan, I remember that after a romantic breakup I felt as if "everyone" was happily coupled off except me. Wherever I went all I saw were twosomes—walking down Fifth Avenue, relaxing in Central Park, shopping in Bloomingdale's—all of them euphoric, while I was on my own.

One day I decided to test this perception and spend an hour or so actually counting the numbers, substituting some statistics for my previous painful perceptions. What did I find? You guessed it! I was far from alone in being alone. The overwhelming number of people I encountered, at least in public venues, weren't part of couples. My initial observation was just an illusion born out of my own sense of loss, especially intense because it was new.

How about posting to yourself that perfection isn't possible? Your own uniqueness is of value. Cherish that and do your best to be who you want to be, but don't compare it to the hype you see online. As for TV or Netflix, it's best to limit yourself to no more than two hours per night. Again, choose quality over quantity. Your time is too precious to waste.

"But," you may be wondering, "I enjoy unwinding over several shows and sometimes binge-watch my favorite series. Why can't I do that?" Excessive screen time, either in front of a computer or TV, can sabotage your efforts to end emotional overeating, especially if you've developed the habit of snacking as you sit. If you're watching the news and it isn't good, as unfortunately has often been the case of late, that will be an extra deterrent to your efforts.

Valuing your time means valuing yourself. If you do enjoy sitting in front of a screen and feel the need to do it for at least an hour or two a night, decide right now that you are going to watch it selectively. Your time is precious. Why fritter it away watching shows that are boring or spend it endlessly channel or web surfing? Choose in advance the show or shows you are going to watch or the activity you will do on the computer. If it isn't entertaining enough to demand your full interest, you will be far more likely to engage in a munch 'n' gulp in an attempt to numb the frustrations of your day. When fully engaged in an activity you'll be less likely to need an additional means of distraction.

In addition, studies show that TV watching lowers your metabolism to the point where it can approach a trance-like state. Even sitting still in a chair or quietly reading renders a higher heart rate! So overdoing tube-time can diminish some of the good work you've been doing by exercising and building fat-burning muscles.

As was mentioned earlier, if you feel you must watch for at least an hour or two a day, one thing that you can do to help minimize snacking is to take up a craft. Yes, it's true that according to some retirement humor the word *craft* is an acronym for "can't remember a f***ing thing!" But for many of us of all ages who love knitting, crocheting, needlepoint, weaving—just to name a few—crafts mean fun, relaxation, great gifts for friends, *and* the ability to wear a small size. (Many Hollywood actresses knit to relax rather than snack between sets!)

Perhaps you'd like to try a craft but don't know where to start. Check out the library for books and magazines on the subject. Ask your friends. Browse at local arts and crafts stores, which offer personal instruction or classes and usually provide easy patterns that are perfect for beginners.

People sometimes chuckle at my knitting, but total strangers often beg me for the pattern of the beautiful glittery stoles I create. Boutiques have offered to buy the result of three or four hours of snack-free time while talking on the phone, watching TV, or standing in line at the post office. In addition, many crafts like knitting are very "centering," almost meditative. Research studies indicate that endorphins similar to those produced by the body while exercising are emitted while knitting, possibly due to the effect that performing a repetitive circular motion has upon the chemicals in the brain.

Perhaps you have children at home, so some of these suggestions seem impractical. What about engaging them in a discussion of "screenless" possibilities for evening entertainment? You may be surprised at the excellent suggestions children have—board games such as classics like Scrabble, or Rush Hour, a more recent favorite, or Charades and Mad-Libs, which are great for larger groups. In addition to helping you cut calories, the time you spend as a family is a precious gift to kids, which can help bring you closer. Just be sure that whatever activity you select is something everyone considers fun, or at least take turns in choosing the activity so that it is usually enjoyable for the whole group.

What other alternatives can you adopt to ensure that your evening is full without food? One of the solutions should not be hard to guess at this point because it may be within view if you're doing what's best for your **SELF**. The **F** is for **F**luids, and filling up on fluids helps us feel more satisfied, as we've discussed earlier. Since it's easy to confuse thirst with hunger, your water bottle should be handy as you read, watch TV, or surf the internet to help you feel hydrated, healthy, and full. This helps combat that empty feeling that leads you to the fridge and calories you would have never consumed if you weren't at home.

Just as you should be sure that whatever activities you select in the evening are special—a special television show that really entertains you and doesn't insult your intelligence, or a special book that involves you—be sure that when you do eat, your snack is equally special. Consider it a designated treat. Your selectivity helps you to guard against mindless, endless munching. Choose your pleasure, feel satisfied, and then finish. The "love it or leave it" scale used in the mealtime techniques is especially applicable here. The strategy to remember is that you will have one small snack or sweet, if you so choose that night, and then stop!

This cutoff point can be a difficult emotional experience for most compulsive overeaters, who frequently experience a sense of mourning similar to the emotions during mealtime when the point of satisfaction is reached and the meal should officially be over. Many clients report an "is this all there is?" kind of disappointment, reflecting an inability to let go of the possibility of finding any additional pleasure from their day. If this rings true for you, don't flee from the feeling. Again, sit down with a piece of paper or your journal. Find the courage to ask yourself, "What steps can I take, even as soon as tomorrow, to make my life more joyful and productive? If I were to picture myself that way, what would I be doing? What would my day be like? How would I know that I was taking the first step in that direction?" You may not find immediate answers, but thinking creatively in this way can start you on the road to making your days more meaningful.

If you continue to find that your evenings seem aimless and you drift toward the kitchen repeatedly hour after hour, you may wish to cut your evenings short. Set your bedtime earlier so that you'll arise at an earlier hour, making it easier to exercise before your other daytime responsibilities begin. By subtly and slowly shifting your biorhythms, you can extend the productive healthy part of your day and limit the time that is destructive to your health. Do this by fifteen-minute increments each week, and in a month or two you'll have an extra edge on getting slim and fit.

There's no doubt that evenings pose a challenge to compulsive over-eaters. Instead of faulting yourself and feeling frustrated—which only serves to fuel your overeating—start to analyze what happens to you at night. Play detective. Pick up clues. Choose your own solutions and see which work best. Remind yourself that every day the sun rises and sets so every day poses another opportunity to learn more about your own evening eating and to do better.

Because this is such a crucial time of day for controlling emotional overeating, we're adding another question for you to ask yourself daily. It's the second part of your one-minute monitor. The first question, as you recall, was, "Am I doing what's best for my **SELF**?" (Remember that stands for—**S**tress, **E**xercise, **L**oving Your Food, and **F**luids.)

The second question derives from a joke I heard many years ago, when a portly individual said, "I'm a light eater. As soon as it gets light, I start to eat." You also need to become a light eater. Not only do you eat lightly, because you savor and love your food, but you are a "light" eater because as the sun goes down, your eating eases up and stops!

After asking yourself, "Am I doing what's best for my **SELF**?," then ask, "Am I a **'light'** eater?" These mnemonic devices are to keep you on track, so be sure to use your one-minute monitor as a reminder, every day, at least once, if not several times. If used well, it will help you remember not only to love your food, but to love life more as well.

As always, our awareness is our greatest strength in helping us to move ahead as we travel toward greater control of our eating and our lives. By looking at our day and asking "Have I managed my stress? Have I exercised enjoyably? Have I loved my food? Have I filled up on fluid and healthy foods? Have I eaten mostly when it's light?," we can come up with clues as to where our strengths lie and what challenges we need to meet.

Then we can pose three strategic enquiries: "What worked well?"; "What proved challenging?"; "How can I plan to maintain what worked and tweak what needs changing?"

The first question, "What worked well?" can be especially helpful. The work of Michele Weiner-Davis—a brilliant, innovative psychotherapist and a founder of Solution-Focused Brief Psychotherapy (SFBP)— has served as an inspiration to me. In her many best-selling books (including *Divorce Busting* and *Change Your Life and Everyone In It*) she advocates the importance of being positive, proactive, and pragmatic—catching others and ourselves when we're doing something *right*!

I will sometimes ask clients at the end of a session to do a homework assignment comprising writing a description of two meals they ate that week—one in which they truly savored their food and the experience and stopped just at the point of satisfaction, and another meal at which they overate and left the table feeling sad and stuffed. At the next session we spend a bit of time analyzing what they can do to correct whatever issues got in the way of their relaxation, enjoyment, and control at the meal that was challenging, but we spend even more time looking at the meal that went well.

So catch yourself whenever you savor a meal and stop just at the point of satisfaction, get out to exercise, manage your stress, and the like. Ask yourself what went *right*—about the situation, your companions (if any), and yourself. If you catch certain elements that seem to work best, ask yourself how you can replicate the scenario and behavior in order to achieve the same successful results repeatedly.

But there's one behavior that has no part at all in helping us move forward as we pursue our efforts. What's that? It's blame. Blame has no place in effectively changing behavior. And as we've seen before, self-hate can serve to both initiate and perpetuate bingeing behavior.

In my early years as a therapist I had the honor of interning at Columbia Presbyterian's New York State Psychiatric Institute, a world-renowned unit where I trained alongside psychiatric residents. Our goal was to help patients who were suffering from severe psychiatric disorders requiring approximately thirty days of in-patient care to return to society functioning as optimally as possible. We also worked with the family members, providing support and helping them, in turn, to offer support to patients.

A phrase I remember from that experience still echoes in my mind because it was our mantra: "You can do better than this." It was accepting yet empowering. It was compassionate yet concerned. It was a statement of fact, and yet a statement of hope.

Why not say this to ourselves when we're off track? It can be powerful.

What's most useful is to consult occasionally with our one-minute monitor as if it were a gentle yet observant friend—the ideally nurturing parent, friend, self from chapter 3. "What happened—or is happening—today?" we might ask ourselves. Checking in several times a day in this way is especially helpful: "Oh, I didn't do anything movement oriented this morning. Is there time for a brisk walk before dinner?" or "I've been working on handling some pain-producing thoughts that have recurred all day, and I know I ate way past a 5 at lunch. Maybe I could get together with a friend for a movie tonight, or go alone, rather than sit home with unstructured time all evening."

That way we can be proactive, rather than reactive, by noticing potential challenges even before they arise. We can also catch patterns in the new behaviors that are happening and those that are not. If we notice that our choices in foods have been less balanced and our portions have been creeping toward super-size rather than sane-size, we can ask ourselves what's contributing to the difference.

One client who hosted guests occasionally noticed that their habits of eating and drinking were contagious. As opposed to the M. F. K. Fisher example above, they ate rapidly, giving little thought to what they were consuming. They also drank heavily and at every opportunity. After checking in occasionally, using our questions, she noticed her tendency to mirror their behaviors, feeling it "unfriendly" to let them eat or drink alone. Eventually a glass of cold water became her new-found friend—something she could cradle, congenial and sober—while they, unfortunately, ate or drank themselves into oblivion.

If certain aspects remain recurrently challenging, another option would be to reread the relevant chapter. Ask yourself, for example, if you've done your best to tune in to pain-producing thoughts that have been plaguing you, or if for some reason you've been choosing to sweep them under the rug.

One client, who came from a family in which she'd been both physically and emotionally abused, realized after time that it felt really strange to feel "good." She experienced discomfort at allowing herself to take pleasure in anything, including food. The very fact that she felt in control was unsettling.

By noticing a pattern of doing well, "What was best for her SELF," and then sliding back, she noted that succeeding made her feel she deserved punishment. She had been taunted by older siblings and her parents whenever she achieved an accomplishment, or strove to do so. "Who do you think you are?," they would say. This insight was truly transformative in allowing her to feel entitled to enjoy both food and life.

So use this method yet again, like an ideal parent or friend within yourself, nurturing and wise, helping you to assess what's working, what's not, and how to move forward to be the best **SELF** for yourself you can be!

8

LOVE YOUR FOOD WITH FRIENDS AND FAMILY

"**W**hat was it like growing up in your family?" That's a question I usually pose to clients at some point in our first session. As our work progresses this often enlarges into an even more meaningful search, leading us to ask ourselves: "In the family in which I was raised, how did I feel about myself? Did I feel free to be me?"

Why is this question so significant? Our ability to make the best choices, ones that will bring us the utmost joy, fulfillment, and health, often rests on how we feel about ourselves and whether we've had the freedom to do what's best for ourselves. And yes, that's often what's best for others in our lives as well. But when we feel constrained by childhood pain to repeat the patterns of the past, doing what's truly best for ourselves is difficult, if not impossible.

This often becomes apparent when I observe clients' ability—or inability—to practice the principles of loving their food when eating with family and friends. What originally was joyfully simple suddenly seems challenging due to concerns about others' reactions and inner rules that are often unconscious, vestigial traces of childhood.

Eva, a fifty-two-year-old married woman who'd been physically and emotionally abused by her mother, finally stood up for herself in a phone call and told her mom that she wouldn't tolerate being spoken to disrespectfully in their weekly conversations. This went very much against her family's rules that she was forbidden to speak up for herself or call out anyone on their abuse. Eva fretted for days about what the repercussions of her outburst would be, emotionally overeating and fearing future punishment. Although her mother's calls became less frequent, Eva did receive support from her siblings and, most important, found new respect for herself.

To gain control of your life and your relationship with food, placing some focus on family is key. Our families of origin helped shape who we are, how we look at the world, and our interactions with others. Only by expanding our awareness can we achieve the insights that will allow us to become who we want to be.

Nancy, a fifty-five-year-old married woman with grown children, snacked compulsively and always kept a great deal of food around the house. She derived much satisfaction from feeding others and feeling she was nurturing them with food. When she looked back, she recalled a childhood of loneliness and isolation.

While it might seem logical to fault Nancy's parents for leaving her alone, causing her to feel abandoned, our goal is to understand, not blame. Only by understanding and accepting our parents' imperfections are we able to embrace our own humanity and the fact that even our best is often flawed.

In Nancy's case, her mother had been an alcoholic. When Nancy, an only child, was at home, not only did she have to do the housework, she needed to help her mother get from the couch to wherever she needed to go for personal care. Her father worked long hours, partly to try to escape the situation at home. Knowing this, it's not surprising that Nancy's childhood was devoid of companionship or joy. Sadly, Nancy's mother had also grown up in a home affected by alcoholism. Her father had been both an alcoholic and physically abusive.

Nancy felt angry and abandoned in her childhood home. Not surprisingly, she wasn't comfortable inviting friends to visit. It was difficult for her to gain a sense of self-acceptance in a household where her mother was both battling childhood memories and attempting to flee from herself. For Nancy, food, rather than alcohol, became the substance she abused as a substitute for the nurturing she'd never had.

Let's first examine your family of origin. Look back to how you felt at mealtime. To what extent did you feel comfortable at the family table? Was there a sense of peace and relaxation? Or was there dread of conflict and anger directed toward others or yourself? Was there a sense of rejection, of not living up to demands and expectations? Were there concerns about being criticized?

Tamara, a single woman in her twenties, grew up in a household where her father slapped her on the face at dinner whenever she said anything of which he disapproved. Although she grew up to become an advertising executive in a prestigious Manhattan firm, Tamara, financially successful at work, struggled with her eating. Her fears that any television spot would be poorly perceived by upper executives often resulted in bingeing behavior, while she berated herself with "shoulds" about what she did or didn't say. Her introjection of her father's disapproval made it hard for her to own her achievements, find joy in dating, and in life. Only by resolving these reactions, created in the past yet carried over into the present, could she reclaim her ability to enjoy life, work, and food.

Misguided actions on the part of parents based on their own narcissistic needs for their children to conform, succeed, or excel can often create a core of self-hate that lasts well into adulthood unless awareness or interventions intrude. As we recall from our earlier work on stress, it takes mourning to work through the loss of not being truly loved for ourselves. The faith to reach out to others and form emotionally corrective experiences with others who love us and whom we love, can, in time, help to heal those early wounds.

Cara, the youngest of three, had two brothers who were out of the house by the time she was twelve. Her mother, who had schizophrenic tendencies, would urge her to take part in schemes that enacted her rescue fantasies for others in the family. Cara, often cornered while alone with her mom at breakfast, felt guilt that she couldn't agree to these plans, often outrageous, on her mother's part and had to endure her mother's rage at her lack of "cooperation." It took many years for Cara to be comfortable with anyone's company at breakfast, and only after forming supportive relationships with friends and eventually a spouse, was she able to set comfortable boundaries for herself in relationships.

None of us had perfect parents, nor are we ourselves perfect. But understanding and, to whatever extent possible, accepting their limitations can help us to truly accept ourselves. Often it's helpful to take our recollections back another generation. Can you remember your grandparents? Equally, if not more important, what, if any, are your parents' remembrances of life as a child? Frequently I hear that clients' parents were *themselves* the children of parents unable to nurture. Clients recall or discover that a grandparent had been the eldest of eight siblings, let's say, and enlisted into childcare at the age of ten, or had lost a spouse suddenly and was left alone with several toddlers to support, or was parented by alcoholics—too emotionally starved to be able to give.

As Theda Salkind, my gifted supervisor at Columbia University Graduate School of Social Work, once said, "You can't expect someone to give a dime if they don't have a dime to give." Extending our search back at least one more generation expands our empathy for our parents and, as a result, ourselves.

Let's return to your experience at the family dinner table. Did you feel as if you and your actions were accepted? Or was there a sense of needing to flee, physically or emotionally, of feeling criticized, unfairly compared, or ignored? Regarding food, were your choices allowed and accepted, or did one or both parents act as either "food pushers" or "food police"? Remembering your experience and reactions can be key in helping you gain a new sense of freedom and control.

In Harriet Braiker's brilliant *The Disease to Please: Curing the People-Pleasing Syndrome*, she spoke of the many "shoulds" that imprison those of us who recognize aspects of ourselves in her title: "As a people pleaser your perceptual antennae are attuned to the needs, preferences, desires, requests, and expectations of others. The psychological 'volume' of other people's needs is turned up high, while the relative volume of your own needs is very nearly muted altogether."[1]

How can we tune in to our own needs at the table—or elsewhere, for that matter—if we're obsessed with satisfying the expectations of others?

Cindy, married, fifty-five, and a homemaker, grew up in a family where her mother, a compulsive dieter, always nagged her about eating the right foods or eating too much. Very little Cindy did at or away from the table could possibly satisfy her parents. Cindy, who struggled to escape a strict dieting mentality yet periodically binged, dared to request a slice of cake for dessert when she and her husband were dining with another couple. She'd envisioned that all four would share, but before she could clarify that, her husband, Herb, interrupted with "What do you need that for?," utterly humiliating Cindy.

Exploring Herb's history, we looked at his youth in a family where he'd always been pressured to be perfect, high achieving in every way. His parents often held him up to his younger siblings as a role model in terms of his schoolwork, but were quick to criticize him whenever he got less than perfect scores in any academic endeavor. Later, they'd often remind him of the sacrifices they'd made for his studies and eventual financial success. Not only did Herb find it impossible to face up to his own imperfections, he was similarly intolerant of family members' flaws. He felt, on some level, personally responsible for his wife's issues with eating—especially when friends and family pressured him with comments like, "Why don't you get her to do something about her weight?"

Taking all of this into account, Cindy knew she needed to initiate a caring, compassionate conversation with Herb, praising him for the loving and caring things he did do in their relationship and recruiting him in her new and healthier approach to eating. This eventually heightened their respect for each other, improving their relationship.

Cindy also had to assert her right to savor just enough of whatever she craved, stopping at the point of satisfaction no matter who was with her or what people said. This marked an important step forward in her personal growth, as she'd previously been constantly conscious of what others thought, whether food was involved or not.

If these concerns feel familiar, ask yourself, "Why do I give away this power? Don't I have the right to decide how to satisfy my needs and find pleasure? Don't I have the right to choose how I feel about myself?" The impact of these questions and our answers extends well past our experiences while eating. Exploring these issues can be crucial in moving forward in self-growth.

Ruth, a widow in her eighties, had a full life with many friends but rarely exercised, in part due to medical issues. Aside from canasta and work for a synagogue group, her main recreation was lunching with friends at elegant restaurants in the area, an activity she engaged in several times a week. After we practiced the *Love Your Food* techniques together, she realized that the entrees she ordered were twice as big as what she needed. Yet she didn't want to bring home half because she knew she tended to ignore the remainder—not considering it novel enough to be appealing later—and it would go to waste. When I suggested she order an appetizer instead of a main course she responded with shock. "I can't do that!" "Why not?" I asked. "Because everyone will think I'm cheap!" she answered.

Ruth's mother had been the eldest of four siblings, a somewhat self-involved woman who had married a wealthy man and lived a financially comfortable life. Her siblings had resented her and often made snarky comments about "the mansion" she lived in or the many vacations she took, hastening the ensuing estrangement between her and her family. Consequently, Ruth, also wealthy, felt compelled to host large parties, lavishing gifts on her sons and their children, as well as friends. While she did this partly for her own pleasure, it was also an attempt to avoid envy, for she believed in superstitions predicting that the evil wishes of the envious came true. It took a good deal of work for Ruth to regain her right not only to eat whatever she wished, or didn't wish to, but also to reclaim her ability to enjoy the good life she had rightfully attained.

Erica, who was in her early twenties when we worked together, suffered from occasional bingeing, often overeating at dinner and then carrying the pattern over into the evenings while she watched TV and/or surfed the internet. Her parents divorced when she was five and she went to live with her father, but when she was twelve he lost his job due to alcoholism and she moved in with her mother. At that point her mother was dating a man who was overly affectionate to her in front of Erica, often at mealtimes. An only child, Erica felt alone, angry, and helpless in these situations, and these feelings carried over to her experience at present-day meals, where she rushed through her food and found it difficult to enjoy the experience. Both at and away from the table she was plagued by perfectionism, taking any minor comment as major criticism and destroying much of the pleasure of her relationships. She often feared abandonment, feeling any imperfection rendered her vulnerable to total rejection. Erica needed to mourn that neither her mother nor father was able to provide her with the nurturing she craved. Only after mourning that loss—and grieving for the sadness of the child she'd once been—could she give herself the love she needed in the here and now, as an adult.

Both friends and family members may be "food pushers"—subtly, or not so subtly, encouraging us by word or example to eat. Recent research shows a strong correlation between our BMI and that of our friends. Whether or not there's some cause and effect, or it's merely an association is debatable. But clearly friends can often synchronize, consciously or not, the amount and types of foods they eat, what they drink, and often seek sameness within a group, especially if one or more of the members have issues.

Halley, a thirty-two-year-old marketing rep, had been sexually abused by a teenaged neighbor who "cared" for her when her parents went out on Saturday night dates, parties, or adult-only trips. Neither parent believed Halley when she told them of the abuse and, given their heavy social schedule, didn't want to relinquish the convenience of the sitter's services. She fled her family to go to college in Miami, but plagued by painful memories and resentments, overate and drank to soothe and distract herself. In her freshman year she gained twenty pounds, which she never took off, and which gradually became forty and started to affect her health.

In college Halley had been the life of the party, and a bit of a class comic. Her sorority sisters loved her funny stories and gags. This carried on as she started her career, as she was often the "star" of the Friday night parties she and her work friends enjoyed.

Eventually she was able to lose the excess weight and adopted healthier habits, like exercise, to keep it off. Although she felt better about herself, her friends complained that she'd been "more fun" before. They found her fun when high but "boring" when sober and eating healthily. She had to face up to their disappointment and realize it was their issue, not hers, so that it didn't sabotage her efforts to take better care of herself.

If this sounds familiar and your friends want you to be their eating, drinking, or smoking buddy, etc., ask yourself this question: "What is his/her/their hidden agenda?"

Since we all share the need to feel good about ourselves, what role does their pressure on you serve to meet this goal? Are they trying to normalize their behavior by surrounding themselves with others doing the same thing to the same extent? By joining them, you may be helping them assuage their guilt and reinforce the illusion "Everyone's doing it! So it must be okay!"

Halley had to fight off powerful urges to comply with her friends' conditions and again be at one with the group. She feared disapproval. Taking a more independent stance and standing up for herself felt "new" and "scary."

Again, ask yourself, "What's the hidden agenda?" Remember that feeling better about themselves—an attempt to preserve or repair their own, perhaps seriously scarred, self-esteem—is often the main motivation.

When Halley and I explored the motivations of her friends it was apparent they had many insecurities of their own. One of her friends was herself obese. Another pal, back in her college days, had an issue with prescription drugs that she tried to hide from all but her closest confidantes. Since her emotional issues interfered with studying, she paid for term papers and had enlisted several sorority sisters to help—a situation she found humiliating. Both now and then, her friends felt less threatened by their own insecurities when Halley acted as an entertainer and took the spotlight off themselves and their own issues. By not doing what was best for herself, she was "enabling" them—and doing everyone involved a disservice.

"How can I handle these comments?" you may be asking. "What do I say when I'm pressured or criticized, or even uncomfortably praised, at meals?"

First, as we've emphasized, reclaim your right to do what, food-wise, feels best and healthiest for you, regardless of the reactions of others around you. Learn what you can from their disapproval and how you react, carrying this information forward for future growth. Second, practice the "sandwich technique" (open-faced and with a plan!) with a friend. This enables you to both finesse the situation and, most important, segue out.

Jessica, a woman in her twenties, appeared very fit but overate at home and exercised to counteract the calories. Since she usually ate salads in restaurants, she was forced to endure her friends' complaints that "she always eats so healthily."

Either a compliment or a brief, lighthearted question could serve as the first "slice of bread" in the sandwich technique response. For example, "Thanks for noticing" and "How observant you are!" are both possibilities, and if that doesn't diffuse the interest, a lightly stated, "Does that bother you?" could serve equally well. The friend might answer, "I know I should eat that way, but just don't have the willpower," to which Jessica might modestly yet self-acceptingly answer, "I'm not perfect, but I'm glad this is one good habit I've developed."

After the compliment, the crux of the message or "meat" is a brief explanatory statement such as "I like eating this way." Or "I've eaten this way so long it's a habit, and I like the light way I feel when I'm finished" or something similar.

The final, and most important, "plan" of your sandwich will serve to get you off the subject, a major objective. "Have you seen the new movie at the Downtown Cinema?" or "I've just finished the greatest suspense novel I've read in a long time. I couldn't put it down once I'd started." You have a right to enjoy your meal. An examination of why, what, and how you eat won't enhance your experience. It will also impair your ability to savor your food until fullness and then to stop.

Those who are critical of how you eat are probably opinionated about how you live, as well. They're probably opinionated about everyone and everything. Remind yourself that you have a right to fully enjoy your food *and* life. If their issues are valid, perhaps you'd like to talk with them about it at another time—away from the table. But don't let the naysayers nix the new habits that are necessary to improve your health!

If you're having trouble sticking to these eating habits when with others, ask yourself an important question, a question trained therapists know to pose whenever a client brings up a symptom that's occurring in one specific situation. "Where else?" In what other scenarios do you find yourself cheating yourself out of what you deserve, sacrificing your own best interests for others, often to your own detriment?

Jillian, a thirty-four-year-old hotel executive, struggled with emotional overeating and excessive weight, a challenge that was complicated by the fact that she worked in an environment where food was often readily available. She'd grown up in a household with a difficult, domineering mother, who expected everyone to bow to her demands and cater to her needs.

Jillian had trouble avoiding the complimentary buffets at work, sometimes scheduling our appointments at times when food was out and available. But she also found it hard to say no to her colleagues, who often asked her for assistance with difficult projects or clients. For a while she resisted my advice to close the door of her office, which would subtly but surely give the message that she was busy and couldn't be disturbed. Only when several of her mentees, young men, were promoted above her, did she start to consider the merits of setting boundaries in this way.

In addition, Jillian was troubled by frequent visits from a cousin who'd come to see their elderly grandmother with four sons in tow, staying with Jillian and expecting to be wined and dined at Jillian's expense. Though divorced and working at a menial job, the cousin managed to treat her sons to expensive sporting gear whenever she came to Florida. Jillian at first had difficulty pointing out the discrepancy of this behavior to her cousin and helping her see the importance of prioritizing her sons' true needs—for school clothes and supplies, for example, rather than for flashy items that they'd soon outgrow. Jillian also had to role-play and communicate the importance of budgeting and spending more wisely, emphasizing that it was what she did in her own life.

It was a struggle for Jillian to regain control of her own life and the right to satisfy her own needs—to learn how to remain sensitive and caring yet not overly self-sacrificing. As Hillel said, "If I'm not for myself who will be for me? But if I am only for myself, who am I? If not now, when?"[2]

This is a balance we all need to find. As the above example shows, being truer to ourselves often results in being there more fully for others. An awareness of ourselves, of our underlying resentments, of what we're doing and why can often result in a better outcome, a true win-win for all involved.

Examine your personal relationships. Explore what's working for you and for those involved, and what's not. Most likely there are positive changes that can be made with better communication and assertive actions on your part. Talking in a way that enables others to hear you is an important tool to make your life less stressful, for you and everyone in it.

Jana, thirty, was excited about her new marriage and moving into her new home. She and her husband had always hoped to return to Florida, where they had grown up, escaping the frigid winters they both hated in the Northeast. They fell in love with the third house they looked at and bought it as quickly as possible, since the seller was entertaining multiple bids. Initially, Jana didn't give much thought to being six blocks away from her mother-in-law, an easy walk, which in no time her mother-in-law started to make on a daily basis. Not only did she come to inspect, she also expected coffee and "a little Danish or whatever you have," which Jana felt obliged to offer. Jana resented the intrusion of these visits and found herself mindlessly overeating from the moment she started on the pastry until well after dinner. She wanted to reclaim her life but didn't know how.

We looked together at ways she could accomplish her objectives. She didn't dislike her mother-in-law, but she wanted their visits to be mutually agreed upon and less invasive. Herself the daughter of a manipulative mother who often played the victim ("Don't mind me, I'm only trying to help!) and a passive father, she had trouble standing up for herself with female authority figures.

We brainstormed through several assertive options. What Jana liked most was, "Marion, I'd love to spend time with you when I have fewer distractions, like the housework and my ringing phone. Let's plan to get together for lunch once a week so that we can have a full hour to sit and chat. There's that new café down the block that we might try first if you'd like. I'll see you next Wednesday, if that day works for you." This took a lot of will-and-won't power on Jana's part, including the need to tell Marion, when she again arrived unannounced, that she'd love to chat but she was running a bath upstairs. Eventually the hint was received and a more mature, respectful relationship resulted between the two.

It's often tough to make these types of tweaks. The annoyance may not always be as obvious as in the example above. So first, tune in to what may need to change. Making effective adjustments in a relationship—before your resentment starts to eat at you, turning to anger, even uncontrollable rage—is the constructive choice. In doing so, which may surprise you, the earliest signs of anger are our friend.

How? Because by spotting resentment before it *eats* at us or, even more literally, before we try to *eat* it away, we can do what needs to be done while we're still in control.

How do we tune in to our resentment? Because my practice is now in Florida, outside my office are palm trees and I often ask clients to look out the windows and notice the breeze. How do they do it? Their eyes automatically go toward the palms, on which they may see a rustling of several fronds, the greenery gently moving in the wind. That, I'll tell them, represents a ten- to thirty-mile-an-hour wind, a relatively peaceful environment, similar to a sense of calmness. If, however, the entire frond was moving, we'd be looking at perhaps a forty- to sixty-mile-an-hour wind, a greater disturbance of the atmosphere, akin perhaps to an annoyance. If the whole tree were starting to sway, the winds would need to be over eighty miles an hour, which would parallel anger, in our emotional analogy. At over a hundred miles an hour, the palm would be in danger, because the trunk might break and the tree might face destruction, an all-too-apt analogy of the disastrous consequences of rage.

Looking at this example, we can sense the necessity of tuning in early, while we're able to think clearly about our options, assertively expressing our needs while taking the needs of others into account. The longer we wait, while not addressing our own escalating emotions, the less able we are to act in a manner that's in our control, rather than merely reacting to the forces we're facing.

Nevertheless, annoyance and irritation, the earliest forms of anger, are our friends, expressing a call for adjustments in our interactions. Like hunger, another helpmate, they're telling us what we need.

What about our children? One of the best gifts you can give them is the role model of a mother or father who loves their family, their life, and food—the latter being one of many pleasures life affords—and of someone who handles stress effectively and away from the table. How many of us reading this would have loved to have had an example like that!

So allow kids many choices, mostly healthy, some just fun, but most important, let them see you savoring your food and stopping at the point of satisfaction, while you tune in to the pleasure of being with them at mealtime. Truly listening to your children while they tell you about their day, showing interest and support, can make for powerful memories. Allowing our children to eat as much or as little as they need—barring extremes that are problematic, of course—is the best way for them to learn how to self-regulate. If you model that behavior at the table, as well as healthy stress management—exercise, assertiveness, and good communication—throughout your day, your children will be lucky.

Consider this ancient Chinese proverb: "Children often cannot hear what we are saying to them because what we are doing screams so loudly." Accepting yourself, even while you work to improve your efforts, and loving your food, yourself, and your family—all send positive messages to everyone else around you.

Before I had my child I resolved never to look into a mirror and say, "Gee, I look fat!" Do you know who really won with that resolution? Me! Not only am I sure it was good for my child, but my own self-image has vastly improved. This resolution helped me to peer into mirrors seeking only the positives, and when we're looking for the good stuff that's all we usually see.

Sadly, the opposite is also true. I've seen many "size zeros" who've come to me saying they're "fat," counting any fold of skin as an imperfection they regard as unallowable. Let yourself accept who you are and how you look, even as you strive to get fitter, healthier, smarter, or whatever! Embracing our present selves as we emerge into people who are even more positive is a wonderful example for our families.

And please, have an "unplugging policy" at the table, if not elsewhere, whenever possible. An anorexic teen I treated fifteen years ago had a mom who was often busy on the phone, planning charity benefits and other events. In spite of the laudable nature of her activities, her daughter felt abandoned and devalued. One of the most therapeutic aspects of "my" therapy with the youngster was the willingness of her dad, a financially successful yet overworked attorney, to drive an hour each way to bring her to see me—unplugged and spending quality time with his daughter.

So respect yourself and those around you—with your time and full attention. The rewards are remarkable.

Since friends are the families we get to choose, ask yourself to what extent you're setting the appropriate example of self-acceptance and mutual respect, and whether they're doing so in return. To what extent do your friends represent who you are, who you were, or who you wish to be? Is it troubling to ask these questions? Possibly so. But that doesn't mean your friends must go. See how they respond to your efforts to move forward. Pals who hinder rather than help you may need to become SDOs (small doses only), at least until they can be brought on board with "I really value your friendship, but blank blank blank upsets me, so can you please do blank, blank, blank instead?" If a warm and assertive request doesn't work, you may need to reevaluate whether your friend is worthy of being called a friend at all.

A final way in which our friends can sabotage our efforts to end our emotional overeating is by example. Recent research shows that as our national BMI enlarges, the number of people attempting to reduce their BMI has shrunk.[3] What's the reason? There are many possibilities, including the fact that traditional weight loss methods, especially strict diets, are odious and ineffective, at best.

But we can't overlook the fact that when everyone in your social network is your size or larger—even though you're aware that your weight is endangering your health—there's a tendency to "normalize" your BMI. A "So what? We're all heavy!" sort of thinking ensues. This can sabotage your strategy to tune in to your hunger, savor only until satisfaction, and then stop.

Linda, a recently retired psychotherapist, prided herself on being a sensitive, caring person, and especially, a good friend. Her parents had also been self-sacrificing to a fault. Many of Linda's friends were heavy and had husbands who admonished them for overeating or choosing "fattening" desserts. When lunching with her friends, she adored the excited look in their eyes whenever she suggested that they order something sweet after the meal. Learning to have only a bite or two, to share the dessert if ordered, or forego it in favor of a tiny treat at another time was hard for her to accomplish. She needed assurance that she was modeling helpful, healthy behavior, and that her friendship would still be valued whether she encouraged "splurging" or not, before she could be "selfish" enough to do what was best for herself.

If any of this feels familiar to you, embrace your new awareness. How you relate to your friends and family, how good you feel about yourself, how free you feel to be your best self, all of these affect your relationship with food.

Notice your setbacks—and your successes—as you continue to move past emotional overeating.

What you achieve may be far more important than you'd ever expected.

9

LOVE YOUR FOOD AT PARTIES AND ON VACATION

Do you feel anxious when you attend a party? If so, you're not alone. Since one of the main reasons that people overeat is to distract themselves from painful thoughts and feelings, let's look at party-related anxiety and how to overcome it.

Here we aren't referring to clinical anxiety, an increasingly common diagnosis in our country today; what we're examining is a less serious but also ubiquitous issue that can impair our ability to fully enjoy social events, our food, and our lives. Be comforted by the fact that you're not alone and let's look together at a few quick pointers to prevent social anxiety.

There are numerous ways to recognize the physiological symptoms of anxiety, including rapid, shallow breathing and overall tension and tightness. Notice these and take some steps to counteract them. Stretching and diaphragmatic breathing (inhaling through your nose and allowing your stomach to expand) can be helpful to alleviate your physical discomfort and help you be more in the moment and relaxed. Some of my clients like to inhale (with their mouths closed) to the count of five and then exhale (with their mouths opened) to the count of eight. Try this and see if it's helpful.

As we learned when we looked at cognitive behavioral therapy, you may be experiencing pain-producing thoughts that are contributing to your anxiety. Thinking, "Wouldn't it be awful" or "terribilizing," if not counteracted, can create anxiety.

Here are some common quandaries many of us face prior to parties.

"What if I overeat?" Parties shouldn't be the only place you see or sample foods you love. If you've ditched your dieting mentality and learned to savor small quantities of your favorite foods, while handling stress in healthier, non-food-related ways, you won't need to fear your proximity to a wide array of tasty treats. In the meantime, make sure to maintain your healthy new habits before and during the party. Get in your daily exercise. Eat your regular, scheduled meals. Thirst can often be confused with hunger, as we've noticed, so drink a bottle of water prior to the gathering and try to keep the caloric and alcoholic beverages you down during the party to a minimum.

"What if no one approaches me?" Then take a risk, reaching out to someone else. A positive comment about the event, the ambience, or the hosts can be an ideal icebreaker. If you choose to comment on someone's clothing or accessories, try to personalize it by saying, "That color looks beautiful on you," rather than just, "I like your dress." That way you're praising not just the choice of attire but the person wearing it.

"What if I have trouble keeping up a conversation?" An effective way to heighten our enjoyment not only of events, but of life itself, is to achieve a state called "flow," first identified by positive psychologists in the late 1970s. If you're an avid exerciser, and hopefully by now you are, you know that it is a "state of total immersion in a task that is challenging yet closely matched to one's abilities."[1] Although the activity here is referred to as a "task," the state of flow is a wonderful feeling that allows us to enter a state of timeless joy.

What's the task of a party? Most of us would agree that we go to these gatherings to have fun and feel good about others and ourselves. So ask questions. Show interest. Take a tip I often share, which I consider one of the best stress antidotes anywhere for any social event. Make it your task to sincerely praise as many people as possible (ideally at least three per party) on something other than their appearance.

Why does this work? Because you only can do this if you really get to know your conversational companion. You must become almost totally immersed in someone other than yourself—in his or her origins, family, interests, and so on—erasing in those moments your ability to be self-consciously concerned about "What is everyone else thinking about me?!"

Who doesn't love to be the object of interest and sincere appreciation? And there's a word for those who extend that to others—*charming*. So go with the flow and have a happier time at the party.

Not only parties, but vacations as well, can pose problems for those of us who tend to overeat emotionally. Ideally, it's all about *experiencing*—being open to the people, the sights, the sounds, the smells, the tastes—when we travel or gather in a group. That's where true satisfaction lies. If we're making our lives as fulfilling as possible, through meaningful activities, managing stress, enjoying myriad pleasures, we don't frantically need to numb ourselves by overeating or indulging in unlawful treats.

HOLIDAY PARTIES

For many people, holidays and holiday parties feel more like work than fun. It's a sad fact, but it's true. Why should this be? Unrealistic expectations may well be partly to blame, as for decades Madison Avenue has barraged us with images of Christmas and Thanksgiving dinners attended by three generations of beautiful, loving family members. And, of course, all the couples are married, blissfully happy, and blessed with 2.3 perfect children.

This phenomenon, a tendency to take stock of our lives, finding fault for any failure to live up to unrealistic or quaint expectations, is wonderfully caricatured on the cover of a hilarious comedy classic—*How to Make Yourself Miserable*. And what were the coauthors wearing on the cover of the first edition? New Year's Eve party hats!

Holiday depression, due to unfulfilled, unrealistic expectations, can be very real and debilitating. And nowhere was this as apparent as at Cancer Care, Inc., a health care agency in Manhattan where I worked for almost eight years. I'd frequently bring this up to the relatives' groups I founded, emphasizing that no one's life is perfect and that when they walked out our doors smiling, anonymously, into the street, the first person they met might also think *their* lives were problem-free.

At that time, the popularity of *When Bad Things Happen to Good People* was at its peak. It's an impressive, impassioned book, but a scholarly, challenging read. Perhaps because of the title, patients' family members were often carrying it—so frequently that it appeared to be the accessory du jour. Clearly, those who loved them wanted to assert that life can be unfair, and that all of us, including the very best among us, are vulnerable.

Unfortunately, many of us get caught up in complicated, seemingly trivial family conflicts during the holidays that greatly interfere with our ability to enjoy both food and family.

Sarah, a sixty-year-old divorcee, was furious that her daughter and son-in-law were inviting her ex-husband and his new wife on Christmas Eve, while her invitation was "only" for Christmas morning brunch. She felt that their time slot was of higher status and that she'd been relegated to a lower tier.

All of her life Sarah had been in competition with her younger sister, who Sarah strongly believed had far more advantages. Sarah envied her sister for being, in her eyes, more attractive, smarter, and their parents' favorite. This resentment poisoned many of her relationships, as friends soon got tired of hearing her bitter complaints about both her sister as well as what she believed to be her daughter's mistreatment.

Not surprisingly, this took a toll on Sarah's health as well, since she'd often overeat while she fumed at all these injustices and often felt too distracted to exercise. Unfortunately, she lost patience with therapy, feeling her complaints weren't getting the acknowledgment they deserved and strongly resisting any new awareness, or perspective, no matter how compassionately these were offered.

It's sad that some of us aren't willing to try something new—a new perspective, a new beginning, opening a new door.

Years ago, single and dateless for New Year's Eve, I heard of a party not far from where I lived. All I knew was the location of the building and the apartment number, not even the name of the host or hostess. Thinking New Year's Eve was perfect for venturing out alone, as anyone else I'd meet who was similarly unaccompanied was probably available, I tucked a bottle of wine under my arm and was on my way. The party was mobbed. Although I never met whoever was hosting, an attractive, sweet guy struck up a conversation soon after I entered. We dated for several years and might have married if he hadn't had his heart set on starting a business in a tiny town in Maine, a locale we both knew would probably not be my scene. But from what I've heard, he became greatly beloved in that town for his unerringly unselfish community-mindedness. I'll always be grateful we met.

So take the risk of heading out alone, whether to a party, a restaurant, or even another country. Whatever you're seeking—solitude or someone else who's special—it's worth it.

VACATIONS

Vacations can be an optimum environment in which to love our food. Ideally, there is minimal stress, magnificent surroundings, and novel, exotic fare. What better place to relax and rehearse the earlier-mentioned **RAFT** techniques? Unfortunately, occasionally reality intrudes.

Recently my husband and I took a three-week vacation to a foreign country, the first organized tour we'd ever tried. The organizing group was highly respected, known for "thinking of everything," and that included gargantuan amounts of food. Although tasty, it was also ubiquitous, copious, and constant.

Some of our cohorts, though quite congenial, subscribed to a syndrome best titled "I paid for it all, so I'm eating it all." Their philosophy seemed to be that because food was there and available, it was their right and their duty to indulge.

Even the rest of us, myself included, took several days to realize we were overeating. At first I ate half of what was offered, but even so I sensed that I was eating a bit past satisfaction. Eventually, I opted to pass up most of what was sent my way. Only after also increasing my exercise did I begin to feel better, lighter, and more like myself.

This belief that more food is better—quantity over quality—may be indicative of a post–Depression era mentality or an emotional residue of dieting and the sense that being on vacation means freedom from strict restrictions. "I paid for it all, so I'm eating it all" exerts a powerful hold over many tourists.

Curt, a sixty-six-year-old accountant, knew he needed to control his emotional overeating, especially since he was semiretired, taking many trips, and often had access to buffets. When food was "free," he always felt it was a bargain. Whenever anything offered was within reach, passing it up seemed somehow wasteful.

Curt's parents came from Germany and had had extensive landholdings until the Nazi regime seized it all—as they did to so many other Jews. After losing their land they fled, initially to Montreal, where

Curt's father set up a business. Extremely frugal, Curt's dad counted every penny he spent, never letting go of anything that might have potential value. Like Curt, he also overate and had been told by his physician that it could cause him health issues, but sadly he never succeeded in gaining control.

Curt had to work through his thoughts that he was being "bad" or "wasteful" by not eating anything and everything available. If there was any obligation that he really needed to abide, it was to remind himself that he owed it to *himself* to take better care of his health. It took a while, but eventually he was able to realize that he could enjoy life more by savoring smaller, saner portions and foregoing extra food. He could also save a good deal of money on medical expenses.

What may be some built-in ways to avoid these vacation pitfalls? Let's take a look at some tips when it comes to planning a trip. Travel plans can be created not only for sightseeing, but for active pursuits, as well. If you love a sport, like skiing, tennis, scuba, golf, or horseback riding, check out opportunities to enjoy these in new environments. Visit the mecca of your sport or interest, a lifelong dream of many enthusiasts.

Wherever you're going, contact the concierge prior to your trip to find out about fitness opportunities available. It often helps to find out whether fitness facilities are on-site, and if so, what types of machines or classes are offered. Once, when visiting a cousin in Walnut Creek, I found a hotel that was actually attached to a gigantic fitness facility, approximately twenty thousand square feet of classes, equipment, racquetball, and more. What an exceptional treat!

Another memorable vacation experience took place near an inn in Newport, Rhode Island, as I returned home from a drive to Maine. Calling ahead and hearing it was near the Cliffside Walk, I awakened early to take the trail. It was truly the most scenic stretch I've ever seen, with megamansions on one side and the Atlantic Ocean on the other— breathtakingly beautiful.

When I was working and living in Manhattan, a perk of the emotionally intense but rewarding work at Cancer Care, Inc., was a six-week vacation. Taking that opportunity to tour Europe, I loosely booked inns and modest hotels, and headed south from Copenhagen to Corvatsch, a peak in the Swiss Alps that reportedly saw fresh snow in August. I'm not sure which was the most fun, skiing an alp in August, or joking with the equipment staff in French as they showed me ski brakes. "C'est pour quand vous tombez," they said. (That's for when you fall.) "Non, *si* je tombe!" I quipped back. ("No, *If* I fall!) And yes, they had a foot of fresh snow the week before.

Not only that, but in summer the neighboring town of St. Moritz was almost empty, and since I was traveling alone, I felt like it was all mine.

So enjoy the totality of your experience whether you're alone or with others. If the thought of entering a party or a restaurant alone still seems scary to you, pretend that you're meeting a friend. And looking at you, who'd know the difference? Ironically, the more comfortable you seem, the more likely you are to be approached, whether you'd prefer to be or not.

Whether you're traveling alone, as a couple, or in a group, remember to plan a plethora of activities—some food related, but mostly of the nongastronomical type. There are obviously many ways to access travel information. The travel guide *Lonely Planet* has been a longtime favorite for insiders' information on many locations.

You might also research the *New York Times 36 Hours In* travel column (available on the internet). Each article focuses on a different city for a select summary of activities, sights, and gourmet eateries. The itinerary easily expands to several more days if time permits, and it's a great way to get ideas about things to do, what to see, and where to eat.

Do your homework in advance. If you plan to be active, you will be. Practicing a wide repertoire of pleasures will make your trip the most memorable.

CRUISE CONTROL

"And what about cruises?" you may ask. "Isn't it inevitable that I'll overeat and hate myself for it when I get home?" No, not if you practice the pointers above, as well as a few that are specific to the cruising experience. Again, plan ahead. Find out about activities offered, fitness classes, lectures, and programs. Pack accordingly, since it's annoying and expensive to buy an item you have at home just to take part in an activity you'd like to try when traveling. (The first things I pack for any trip are my sneakers and workout wear.)

At mealtimes, it's the experiences—food among them—that truly make a trip memorable. Get to know those around you, enjoy the sights, as well as the sensations surrounding your food, and enjoy the totality of your experience. Be sure to keep your **RAFT** techniques—**R**elaxation, **A**wareness, **F**ullness Check, and **T**aking Charge of the Moment—in practice. Elegant surroundings and excellent food can make it even easier. Feast your eyes on the décor, the views of the ocean, the appearance and attire of those around you. Savor it all.

"But what about the midnight buffet?" you might ask. "Isn't that guaranteed to bring on a binge?" Yes, the notorious midnight buffet (now often starting as early as six in the evening) is often described as the downfall of dieters. But you're not a dieter! In fact, if you've been following the suggestions so far, you've probably had such a great morning class at the gym—yoga or Zumba or spin or whichever—engaged in so many interesting activities, and made the acquaintance (if not friendship) of so many fascinating fellow passengers, that you're in bed sound asleep before midnight.

If you do make the buffet, here are some pointers so you can enjoy the experience without regret:

- *Sip.* Have a glass of water. Since hunger and thirst are easily confused, you may find that a beverage is all you want or need. Or at most you might want one bite of something with your coffee or tea.
- *Survey.* Check out every table to see what's offered. Since you're going to have just a little, you'll want that to be something special you really desire.
- *Sample.* Take a tiny plate and try a teaspoon-sized sample of anything you aren't sure you'll like. Why put it on your plate if it doesn't please you?
- *Select.* Choose one or two very small tastes of whatever appeals to you. Check your fullness as you do. You're probably not hungry (which would be at less than a 5), so a tiny taste should be enough to satisfy your curiosity.
- *Sit.* Now that you've made your selection, relax and socialize.
- *Savor.* Notice your surroundings, both animate and inanimate. Note the look, taste, texture, and scent of whatever you chose.

Even the tiniest portion, a tablespoon or two, is memorable if we truly treasure it.

- *Stop.* Tomorrow is another day. You'll want to be up early to be active and take advantage of the many options offered—including a healthy breakfast that will be so much more appealing if you don't overeat now.

Again, this is a pleasure-oriented—quality, not quantity—approach. And yes, everyone should experience the midnight buffet at least once, but probably not more often than that. Who really requires a lot of food after dinner late at night? For most of us, it isn't even appealing. We've been satisfied earlier and now we want to sleep—and sleep well.

Perhaps you feel you have to go—"It's a happening. It's something worth seeing, if only once." But notice, and this may seem unkind, the appearance of those around you. Many of the midnight buffet mavens may not look nearly as fit and healthy as you'd like to be.

Another, more simple strategy is to go with friends and split one piece of pie or cake two, three, or four ways. One health-oriented restaurant chain in my community serves dessert in champagne-size goblets—a sane-size serving that works for me!

As many of the meals on a cruise may be buffet style, try adding the first four Ss to your mealtime strategy—*Sip, Survey, Sample,* and *Select.* Use one small dish for salad, a cup for soup, and another small dish for your entrée. Once you've sat down, resort to your **RAFT** techniques as you've practiced before. Be sure to remember your Fullness Check, as you may not want as many courses as you think.

If those around you are overeating, you may be prone to synchronize and overindulge as well. Awareness is key. If you sense this is happening, take back control. Get some coffee, tea, or another noncaloric beverage if you'd prefer to continue a conversation, or politely excuse yourself and enjoy some non-food-related fun.

On land or on sea, doing what's best for your **SELF**, and staying a *light* eater—in other words, using your one-minute monitor—will keep you on track. And remember, if you're doing it right, you'll enjoy your trip more!

10

LOVE YOUR FOOD FOR A LIFETIME

Ideally you're enjoying this plan, wish you'd always eaten this way, and hope you always will. But as we discussed in our chapter on stress, changes can be challenging, even good ones. As we adapt to life, we can sometimes lose hold of even the happiest and healthiest new habits. But don't forget that awareness is key. Our lapses are precious in helping us pinpoint potential stressors and how we're prone to react. They're valuable assets in our learning and growth. So say, "Thank you, lapse!" and learn.

Karen, a fifty-five-year-old married woman, had a dear friend who was coping with the final stages of advanced cancer. Karen called often and sometimes texted, especially when her friend was too weak to talk. The husband of her friend, however, spying these texts, was furious that both women were referring frankly to the illness and its possible aftermath. He barred his wife from any further contact with Karen, which, because of his wife's weakened condition, she allowed.

Although loving her food, and following this plan until this period, Karen then began to overeat, blaming herself for the honesty of her messages, and feeling guilty about intruding. Although ambivalent about sending those messages, she sensed that her friend welcomed her honesty. Examining her practices, Karen realized that it was stress that was undermining her resolve and that she was eating in the evening as she dwelled on what she felt she "should" be doing to help her friend.

Karen had to combat her self-blame, realize that others can be threatened by real feelings, and acknowledge her excellent intentions before she was able to regain control of both her food and her life. Eventually her relationship with the couple was reestablished and she was able to again provide comfort and support to someone who was like a sister.

Mitch, forty-five, married with two teenagers, likewise dealt with stress due to the illness of a loved one. His father, hospitalized for several weeks, was eventually discharged to a nursing home, in part because Mitch didn't have the room in his home to accommodate him and full-time help.

Always a difficult man, Mitch's dad became more irritable as he aged. He often reminded Mitch of the many sacrifices he'd made for him and that Mitch's brothers, one in California and the other in England, were more successful. Although Mitch visited twice a week, whenever he prepared to leave, his father would say, "Leaving so soon? I'm sure you just can't wait to go." This irritated Mitch to no end, especially since it reminded him of the nastiness with which his dad used to treat Mitch's mother.

Mitch, simmering with anger, and resorting to negative name-calling and shoulds while he ate, would then overeat at dinner and thereafter. Only by doing his daily monitoring, noticing to what extent he was on and off track with managing stress and his eating, could he be conscious of this backsliding.

We spoke at length of Mitch's frustration with his dad, and how it affected his ability to feel good about himself and take care of his health. Mitch had to mourn the fact that this disapproving, unhappy man, who'd turned away all other means of emotional support due to his bad behavior, was the only father he had and had ever known. He needed to be helped to feel good about the man and the father he'd himself become, in spite and perhaps because of this negative role model. We can sometimes learn from a "don't" in spite of the pain.

Eventually, Mitch was able to say, "I love you, Dad, and I want to come, but it hurts me when you blame me for returning to my family. Please try to stop, because I want to be able to enjoy my visits more." Mitch had to say this several times, and even skip a visit one week, until his dad finally got the message

Savannah, a forty-two-year-old corporate marketing executive, was excited about a promotion. She quickly learned, though, that one of the perks of being next in line to the CEO of a major company was the receipt of texts 24/7, holidays included!

Prior to this, Savannah had gained control of her emotional overeating, which usually occurred in the evenings. Eventually, though, the stress of constantly being on call to her boss started to get to her. Not only did she binge, but she felt sick physically, suffering with symptoms of chest pain and indigestion, rarely feeling well. Once cleared by her physician, she finally realized she had to reclaim her life.

We worked together on assertiveness techniques, finally finding a suitable strategy. Savannah was able to say to her boss, "I tend to work better when I have time to refuel. When I take a brief break to regroup I come up with my best ideas." Although at first reluctant to hold back on her requests, eventually Savannah's boss became more reasonable, and after a while she confided that her own family appreciated that she seemed more present.

Both she and Savannah needed to learn an important skill, one that's crucial in my field and many others—to compartmentalize. If we exit work dwelling on unfinished business or unresolved issues of our clients, we can wear ourselves out both emotionally and physically, rendering ourselves unfit to do our best on an ongoing basis. We need to learn to let it go. We're not going to find an answer at the dinner table, or as we lie in bed trying to sleep, and trying to force it will prevent us from operating at optimal efficiency the next day. Very often, however, after taking a break from concentration, a serendipitous solution appears.

Whether it's eustress or distress that's taking you off track, try to tune in to what's changed in your life, how you're reacting and how that can be improved. In Savannah's case, she'd had a critical mother who never felt Savannah did enough for her. Modifying her boss's requests meant being a "bad girl," a label that brought punishment to her as a child. She had to acknowledge her strengths, including impressive professional accomplishments, in order to take charge.

Another client, Hillary, in her twenties and newly married, took great pride in her career. Fired for the first time in her life, she felt traumatized. Though her eating had been in control prior to the incident, afterward she felt depressed and spent a lot of time at home, munching on whatever she could find. Through self-monitoring, she saw that she'd become anything but a "light" eater and wanted to work on this reversion.

We spent a lot of effort tackling her resistance to job hunting. Her husband was capable of being their sole financial support since he was successful in his field but that hadn't been their plan and he was starting to feel resentful. After exploring a number of online options, she spotted a local networking event that was open to people of all professions. Still, she was reluctant to go. Fearful of entering the room alone, she found none of my strategies helpful. Finally, I offered something unconventional. If she'd feel more comfortable, I'd even go to the meeting myself so that she'd feel she "knew" someone in the room, never, of course, letting anyone know our relationship.

As she considered this option, she came to a session bringing this dream. She'd been standing on an ocean liner, an elegant vessel that was docked in port. A woman on deck—coincidentally my age, same height and hairdo—took, to Hillary's horror, a fatal leap off the bow of the boat.

What did this dream have to tell us? We looked at the elements. First, I always encourage clients to explore the feelings in their dream. While her perch on the boat seemed safe, she felt frightened by the leap she saw in front of her. The boat was docked and to Hillary that seemed indicative of her own stagnation. My presence in the dream could represent a part of her that wanted to move forward but was frightened. My fatal leap suggested to her that pressing forward was, in fact, perilous. Although at first resistant to the direction of the dream, she later became thoughtful as we looked at her fears of rejection; her father's critical attitudes; the painfulness of her parents' divorce, in which she was forced to take a side; and how hard it was for her to face anything less than excellence in any aspect of her life.

Our goal was to help her accept her efforts and give herself credit for trying her best, whatever the outcome. Life would go on, whatever the results of her interviews. Her self-confidence could survive even if she wasn't immediately successful in securing a new position. Several weeks later, Hillary ended our sessions, leaving me wondering whether she'd succeeded in her objectives. A month or so later, when I was out at dinner, she and her husband approached, smiling, and thanked me. She had faced her fears, found new employment, and moved forward.

What is one of my greatest joys in being a therapist? It's seeing my clients transform themselves into the people they've always wished to be. It's the sheer enchantment of watching people who'd been hindered—by doubts, fears, anxieties, self-hate, and other setbacks—slowly but surely move forward. Sometimes I hear about triumphs, as clients tell me they've tried something new or different that they'd never have been able to accomplish before. I may notice a deeper, clearer tone of voice, and less hesitation in speaking. Or the evidence may be visible in a more erect posture and a gaze that's more direct and self-confident.

If emotional overeating has been a main issue, they report their success in feeling more in control around food—in stopping at satisfaction, leaving food uneaten on their plates, foregoing snacks and other unnecessary items that were offered to them when they weren't hungry. They feel proud that they've taken charge of their eating and their lives.

What's unfortunate about using food as an attempt to cope with stress is the stagnation inherent in relying on one static, ineffective defense throughout the years. By relying on food and food alone to soothe ourselves, assuage our pangs of loneliness, momentarily dissipate despair—*to distract ourselves from painful thoughts and feelings*—we perpetuate a static, helpless, unhealthy state. This self-induced helplessness renders us unable to be aware of what we, ourselves, are doing to contribute to our pain, and, most important, how we can minimize it or manage it and *move* forward.

Again, awareness is often the key to unlocking the mystery of why we're trapped.

Hannah, a twenty-five-year-old teacher, had been dating her boyfriend for three years. Although unsure of whether he was Mr. Right, she recognized he had many good qualities and was hesitant to let him go. In the past, when they had disagreements about his punishing work schedule—he was a busy resident—and his guilt that he didn't have enough time to spend with her, she would retreat and overeat. She always felt terrible afterward, even more alone and unlovable than she'd felt beforehand.

Her previous pattern, developed since her teen years of dating, had been to assume lack of interest whenever any misunderstandings or differences arose. She'd then withdraw, eat, and either end the relationship herself or see it die.

Her parents had divorced suddenly, when her father had an affair with an assistant at work. The community had been aware of the scandal and it was humiliating for both Hannah and her brother, as her father was well known and highly respected in their town. The loss of self-esteem she experienced then seemed to follow throughout her life, as she felt rejected whenever there were any questions raised about any aspect of her relationship with a man.

Together we explored how frozen she felt in that state of helplessness she'd felt as a child. While unable at six years old to revise her relationships, as a more mature young woman, she could modify her life and make modifications.

Hannah had been doing well in our work and was ready to "graduate out" until her boyfriend requested a "talk." She realized in our session that she feared abandonment and was reverting to feelings of helplessness and guilt that she'd known earlier. By tracking her behavior she noticed not only these feelings of anxiety but changes in behavior, as her choices in foods had reverted to only those that tasted sugary, cold, and sweet. She seemed to be seeking a childlike solace in food, mainly ice cream and candy, rather than facing her real-life conflicts as the mature and competent woman she'd become.

Working together we helped her to break out of this cycle of mindless eating, self-imposed self-hate, and withdrawal. She decided to speak with her boyfriend more openly about her expectations of the relationship and that she wasn't as needy for his time as he'd assumed. She also decided to conform more to his schedule, planning dates around time slots that worked for him, even if the hour or day didn't conform to a "Saturday night, pick you up at eight" expectation.

This worked out better for both of them. He felt more rested and was able to be more engaged and loving. He was also appreciative of her selflessness and flexibility. Hannah used the time to develop new skills and planned to add some additional technology to her classroom and embark on some online artwork as a creative outlet for herself.

Not just distress, but eustress, can be troubling, as we discussed in earlier chapters. It can heighten our expectations of ourselves, which, if unrealistically high at the start, will then soar into the stratosphere. When expectations fly that high, there's only one way to go—downward into depression.

Heather, a thirty-eight-year-old, married, midlevel executive, had been hoping for a promotion for many years and had been considered for several. She'd always been passed up, sometimes hurtfully. In one instance an email circulated saying she'd been cut from a group of three other candidates. So it came as a shock when a new opportunity opened up, with a new upper-management team at the helm, and she won the promotion. This new position was the dream job she'd aspired to for a lifetime. Yet in spite of having "won" the new position, Heather was surprised at how unhappy and stressed she felt. Though not totally unexpected, the envy of her colleagues was uncomfortable. And her husband's lack of enthusiasm about her achievement was unsettling. But what absolutely terrified her was the possibility that she couldn't perform—and not just outstandingly, but even adequately.

Almost nothing that had previously brought her pleasure—food, sports, even spending time with the people she loved—seemed to be helpful. Aware, due to her daily monitoring, that she was eating past fullness yet not enjoying food, exercising only sporadically, and feeling perpetually stressed, she knew she needed to take action.

Heather was suffering from a full-blown case of *The Imposter Phenomenon*, referring to the title of the ever-popular classic by Dr. Pauline Rose Clance. It's a syndrome that's unfortunately far too common, especially among women, who often feel that they're frauds and they don't deserve their status at work, or at home, unless they're absolutely perfect at everything they do. Such people find it very hard to own their success; their ability; and, most important, their right to enjoy life.

Does this sound in any way like you? Have you agonized endlessly, blaming yourself for an actual or imagined mistake? Equally unfortunate, have you avoided the risk of attempting a new and exciting project due to a fear of "messing up"—making an error and experiencing the consequences? Perhaps you've put off doing work that could have been enjoyable if only you'd done it on time, rather than procrastinated.

All of us feel these fears at times. But ask yourself, "Are these concerns keeping me from truly living and loving my life?" If you hesitate to answer, you may be onto something. Fortunately, there's an answer that can free you from your fear and allow you to move forward.

Perhaps you've heard this saying: "The perfect is the enemy of the good." It may be ancient and, in fact, its exact origins are unknown. Perhaps it was Voltaire who first referred to this concept. Maybe Shakespeare. But what's apparent is the truth that has resonated with so many for so long.

Do you relate to the wisdom within this statement? Too many of us are overly self-critical, using grades of either an A+ or an F on aspects of our lives, who we are, and how we look, rather than learning to love the liberating mind-set of B+ or A– living.

So drop the duel between "perfect" and "good" when you evaluate your efforts.

"Perfectly good" is good enough.

If you're truly perfectionistic this will totally turn you off. "She's telling me to be mediocre!" you're thinking as you refuse to relent.

What's so wonderful about this perfect and good détente, this win-win approach between two adjectives?

- *Perfectly good* projects get started and tweaked as required as they're in progress.
- *Perfectly good* assignments are completed and handed in on time without undue anxiety and stress. The professor or employer involved is often very appreciative of the promptness.
- *Perfectly good* relationships are begun and explored. These either endure or end, so that the lessons learned can be put to work within them or with future partners.
- *Perfectly good* interests are pursued and can lead to new social networks and great times whatever the skill level at which they're performed. Freed from perfectionism, possibilities expand, life looms large, and fear fades.
- *Perfectly good* choices and efforts afford us self-satisfaction rather than self-hate.
- *Perfectly good* efforts at loving our food and improving our health are tweaked as needed, so we learn and grow and our lives can improve.

Try it and see how it feels. My guess? *Perfectly good!* This is an advantage of coming back home to the techniques we've learned. It feels good.

Returning to the relaxation of taking some breaths, sitting back and stretching, tuning in to ourselves and our bodies, savoring not only our food but our surroundings—all afford us a refreshing revisit to times of less stress, a reminder of how we can feel and would like to feel again.

Return without recrimination but with new knowledge of what took you off track and how to stay on course continuously.

Remember your one-minute monitor and your eating techniques, and remember to learn new fun ways to love yourself, your food, and your life. Don't be dismayed at disappointments—whatever they may be. Love your lapses. Embrace them. They're sending you a gift—that of helping you learn and grow and better achieve what's truly best for you!

I've enjoyed our journey together. I hope you have, too.

All my best wishes as you move forward!

RESOURCES

Eating Disorder Organizations

Alliance for Eating Disorders Awareness
    www.allianceforeatingdisorders.com/portal/
    866-662-1235
National Eating Disorders Association (NEDA)
    www.nationaleatingdisorders.org
    800-931-2237
National Institute of Diabetes and Digestive and Kidney (NIDDK)
Health Information Center
    www.niddk.nih.gov/health-information
    800-860-8747
Oliver-Pyatt Centers
    www.oliverpyattcenters.com
    866-511-HEAL
Renfrew Center
    www.renfrewcenter.com
    1-800-RENFREW

NOTES

INTRODUCTION

1. Rachel X. Weissman, "Getting Bigger All the Time," *American Demographics*, February 1999.

2. Pew Research Center, "Eating More; Enjoying Less," *Social & Demographic Trends*, April 19, 2006, http://www.pewsocialtrends.org/2006/04/19/eating-more-enjoying-less/.

3. Centers for Disease Control and Prevention, "Obesity and Overweight," National Center for Health Statistics, last updates May 3, 2017, https://www.cdc.gov/nchs/fastats/obesity-overweight.htm.

I. "LOVE MY FOOD?!"

1. Tal Ben-Shahar, *Happier* (New York: McGraw-Hill, 2007), 42.

2. Theodore I. Rubin, *Compassion and Self-Hate* (New York: Ballantine, 1977), 111.

2. DIETS DO WORK—TO CAUSE COMPULSIVE OVEREATING AND BINGEING!

1. Charlotte N. Markey, "Don't Diet," *Scientific American Mind* (September/October 2016), 48. doi:10.1038/scientificamericanmind0915–46.

2. "Obesity. Is It an Eating Disorder?" ANRED, accessed October 1, 2017, https://www.anred.com/obese.html.

3. Ibid.

4. Charles Duhigg, *The Power of Habit: Why We Do What We Do and How to Change It* (New York: Random House, 2012), 19.

5. Roxane Gay, *Hunger: A Memoir of (My) Body* (New York: HarperCollins, 2017), 17.

3. POINT #1: STRESS—LEARN FROM IT TO LESSEN IT

1. Alice Miller, *Prisoners of Childhood* (New York: Basic Books, 1981), 85.

2. Hans Selye, *The Stress of Life* (New York: McGraw-Hill, 1984), 74.

3. Karen Horney, *Neuroses and Human Growth* (New York: W. W. Norton, 1950), 64–85.

4. Robert Chernin Cantor, *And a Time to Live* (New York: Harper Colophon Books, 1978), 33.

5. Ann S. Kliman, *Crisis: Psychological First Aid for Recovery and Growth* (New York: Holt, Rinehart and Winston, 1978), 6.

6. Ibid.

7. Colin Murray Parkes, *Bereavement* New York: International Universities Press, 1998), 85–86.

8. Elisabeth Kübler-Ross, *Questions and Answers on Death and Dying* (New York: Macmillan Publishing, 1974), 25–26.

4. POINT #2: EXERCISE—LEARN TO LOVE IT

1. Centers for Disease Control and Prevention, "National Diabetes Statistics Report, 2017" (Atlanta, GA: Centers for Disease Control and Prevention, U.S. Dept. of Health and Human Services, 2017).

2. "Increased Physical Activity Associated with Lower Risk of 13 Types of Cancer," National Institutes of Health, May 16, 2016, https://www.nih.gov/news-events/news-releases/increased-physical-activity-associated-lower-risk-13-types-cancer.

3. Merrill Fabry, "Fitness throughout the Ages," *Time*, April 28, 2017.

4. Centers for Disease Control and Prevention, "Physical Activity and Health: A Report of the Surgeon General Executive Summary" (Atlanta, GA: Centers for Disease Control and Prevention, U.S. Dept. of Health and Human Services, 1996).

5. Centers for Disease Control and Prevention, "Current Physical Activity Guidelines," last modified November 29, 2016, https://www.cdc.gov/cancer/dcpc/prevention/policies_practices/physical_activity/guidelines.htm.

6. Centers for Disease Control and Prevention, "Target Heart Rate and Estimated Heart Rate," last modified August 10, 2015, https://www.cdc.gov/physicalactivity/basics/measuring/heartrate.htm.

7. Eric Finkelstein et al., "Effectiveness of Activity Trackers with and without Incentives to Increase Physical Activity (TRIPPA): A Randomized Controlled Trial," *The Lancet: Diabetes and Endocrinology* 4, no. 12 (December 2016): 983–95, doi:10.1016/S2213–8587(16)30253–4.

8. Ibid.

9. John M. Jakicic et al., "Effect of Wearable Technology Combined with a Lifestyle Intervention on Long-Term Weight Loss: The IDEA Randomized Clinical Trial," *JAMA* 316, no. 11 (September 20, 2016): 1161–71, doi: 10.1001/jama.2016.12858.

10. Elizabeth A. Richards, Niwaka Ogata, and Jeffrey Ting, "Dogs, Physical Activity, and Walking (Dogs PAW)," *Health Promotion Practice* 16, no. 3 (2014): 362–70, doi:1177/1524839914553300.

11. Edward T. Creagan, *How Not to Be My Patient* (Deerfield Beach, FL: HCI, 2003), 251.

12. Edwin C. Bliss, *Getting Things Done* (New York: Bantam Books, 1976), 53.

13. Hana Kahleova et al., "Meal Frequency and Timing Are Associated with Changes in Body Mass Index in Adventist Health Study 2," *Journal of Nutrition* (July 2017), doi:10.3945/jn.116.244749.

5. POINT #3: LOVE YOUR FOOD—HANDS-ON TECHNIQUES

1. Edwin C. Bliss, *Getting Things Done* (New York: Bantam Books, 1976), 69–70.

6. POINT #4: FLUIDS AND HEALTHY FOODS—LEARN TO LOVE THEM

1. Roberta Larson Duyff, *American Dietetic Association Complete Food and Nutrition Guide* (Boston: Houghton Mifflin, 2012).

2. Tammy Chang et al., "Inadequate Hydration, BMI, and Obesity among US Adults: NHANES 2009–2012," *Annals of Family Medicine* 14, no. 4 (July 2016), doi:10.1370/afm.1951.

3. "Water Intake Overlooked in Obese Individuals," University of Michigan, Family Medicine, July 15, 2016, https://medicine.umich.edu/dept/family-medicine/news/archive/201607/water-intake-overlooked-obese-individuals.

4. Jennifer Drawbridge, "Can Water Help You Lose Weight?" *Cooking Light*, July 11, 2016, http://www.cookinglight.com/healthy-living/water-can-help-you-lose-weight.

5. Carroll A. Lutz and Karen Rutherford Przytulski, *Nutrition & Diet Therapy: Evidence-Based Applications* (Philadelphia: F.A. Davis, 2005), 168.

6. Silvia Maier, Todd Hare, and Aidan Makwana, "Acute Stress Impairs Self-Control in Goal-Directed Choice by Altering Multiple Functional Connections within the Brain's Decision Circuits," *Neuron* 87 (August 2015), doi:10.1016/j.neuron.2015.07.005.

7. James Hamblin, *If Our Bodies Could Talk* (New York: Doubleday, 2016), 147.

8. Lisa Esposito, "DASH: The Best Diet with the Least Buzz," *U.S. News & World Report*, February 6, 2015, https://www.health.usnews.com/health-news/health-wellness/articles/2015/02/06/dash-the-best-diet-with-the-least-buzz.

9. "DASH or Mediterranean: Which Diet Is Better for You?" Harvard Health Publishing, August 2015, https://www.health.harvard.edu/diet-and-weight-loss/dash-or-mediterranean-which-diet-is-better-for-you.

10. Barbara Rolls and Robert A. Barnett, *The Volumetrics Weight-Control Plan: Feel Full in Fewer Calories* (New York: HarperTorch, 2005), 102.

11. David A. Kessler, *The End of Overeating: Taking Control of the Insatiable American Appetite* (New York: Rodale, 2010), 14–15.

12. Dairy Council of California, "Serving-Size Chart," HealthyEating.org, accessed 25 September 2017, https://www.healthyeating.org/Portals/0/Documents/Schools/Parent%20Ed/Portion_Sizes_Serving_Chart.pdf?ver=2017-08-31-150411-207.

13. *American Medical Association Complete Guide to Prevention and Wellness* (Hoboken, NJ: Wiley, 2008), 4.

14. "The Truth about Fats: The Good, the Bad, and the In-Between," Harvard Health Publishing, last modified August 22, 2017, https://www.health.harvard.edu/staying-healthy/the-truth-about-fats-bad-and-good.

15. Center for Science in the Public Interest, "10 Best Foods," *Nutrition Action Healthletter*, March 8, 2016, https://cspinet.org/eating-healthy/what-eat/10-best-foods.

7. POINT #5: EVENING EATING—"ARE YOU A 'LIGHT' EATER?"

1. Julie-Ann Amos, "Acid Reflux (GERD) Statistics and Facts," Healthline.com, June 30, 2012; "Digestive Diseases Statistics for the United States—National Diseases Information Clearinghouse (n.d.), Home- *National Digestive Diseases Information Clearinghouse,* March 5, 2012, https://www.niddk.nih.gov/health-information/health-statistics/digestive-diseases#specific.

2. M. F. K. Fisher, *The Art of Eating* (Hoboken, NJ: Wiley, 2004), 512.

8. LOVE YOUR FOOD WITH FRIENDS AND FAMILY

1. Harriet B. Braiker, *The Disease to Please: Curing the People-Pleasing Syndrome* (New York: McGraw-Hill, 2001), 51.

2. M. Pirkei Avot 1:14.

3. Cari Nierenberg, "Unhealthy Trend: Fewer Americans Are Trying to Lose Weight," *Livescience,* March 7, 2017, https://www.livescience.com/58145-fewer-americans-are-trying-to-lose-weight.html.

9. LOVE YOUR FOOD AT PARTIES AND ON VACATION

1. Jonathan Haidt, *The Happiness Hypothesis* (New York: Basic Books, 2016), 1995.

INDEX

abuse, 119–120, 121

acceptance: of change for stress management, 32–34; of feelings, 30–31, 109; of parents' imperfection, 120; of parents' limitations, 121–122. *See also* self-acceptance

activities: as alternatives to evening eating, 113–114; for enjoyment, 23, 23–24; exercise, 63–67; exercise group, 53, 67; vacation planning of, 138, 138–139, 139, 139–140

addictions, 84

aerobics, 58; benefits, 62; CDC on, 59–60; endorphins from, 58

American College of Sports Medicine, 59

American Demographics, ix–x

American Dietetic Association's Complete Food and Nutrition Guide (Duyff), 88

Americans: relationship with food, 2; SAD for, 92, 101; weight loss in relation to, ix

anecdote: on abuse, 119–120, 121; on apology, 48–49; on awareness of feelings, 109–110; on boundaries, 121, 127–128; on communication, 47–48, 128–129; on compartmentalization, 144–145; on compassionate conversation, 122–123; on compulsive eating, 4; on depression, 29, 41; on dreams, 25, 145–146; on eating awareness, 17–18; on exercise

motivation, 55; on exercise program, 57–58, 58; on expression of feelings, 81; on fear of being a fraud, 149; on fear of disapproval, 125–126; on frugality, 137–138; on frustration with family, 144; on habit changing, 7; on holiday resentment, 136; on hydration, 89; on lack of nurturing during childhood, 120; on pain-producing thoughts, 46–47; on perfectionism, 124; on postdiet defiance, 16–17; on relationship self-esteem, 147–148; on sandwich technique, 126–127; on seizing present moment, 8; on self-acceptance, 123–124; on self-accusations, 39, 80–81; on self-blame, 143–144; on self-denial, 117–118; as teaching tool, x

anger: childhood as source of, 80; with family, 144; as friend, 129, 130; after mealtime, 78, 80

Anorexia Nervosa & Related Eating Disorders (ANRED), 13

anxiety, 133

apology, 48–49

The Artist's Way (Cameron), 23

assertiveness, 49

athletes, 94

awareness: anecdote on eating, 17–18; anecdote on feelings, 109–110; for behavioral change, 3, 110–111; during

ABOUT THE AUTHOR

Arlene B. Englander, LSCW, MBA, has been a Columbia University-trained, licensed psychotherapist for more than twenty years. She also completed an MBA at New York University. Currently in private practice throughout North Palm Beach, Florida, she specializes in treating persons coping with eating disorders, relationship issues, depression, anxiety, grief, and stress. *Love Your Food®*, her nondieting, psychologically oriented program for compulsive overeaters and bulimics, has been featured on "Health Beat" on a South Florida CBS TV affiliate and has been presented in seminars at local hospitals, health clubs, and organizations. She has been a frequent guest on 960 AM/FM Radio and a frequent contributor to the advice column for *Simply the Best*, a local magazine with thirty-six thousand subscribers.

Englander developed many of her theories about stress management while working at Cancer Care, Inc., which counsels thousands of patients and families dealing with advanced cancer. She subsequently developed stress management programs for use in hospitals, law firms, and other settings. As director of Community Education at the Holliswood Hospital, a private psychiatric hospital in New York City renowned for its eating disorders program, her responsibilities included the production of educational seminars attended by as many as five hundred psychiatrists, psychologists, social workers, psychiatric nurses, and guidance counselors. While on staff at Lenox Hill Hospital and American Express Travel Related Services, she was also involved in developing health promotion programs.

She is currently on the Steering Committee of the Palm Beach County Unit of the National Association of Social Workers, which is actively involved in bringing educational programs and other events to clinical social workers in the community.

Aside from her professional training and experience, Englander is also personally familiar with the issue of eating disorders, since she is a former emotional overeater.